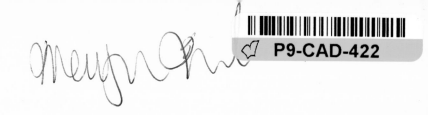

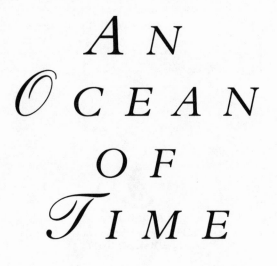

AN OCEAN OF TIME

Alzheimer's:
Tales of Hope and Forgetting

PATRICK MATHIASEN, M.D.

SCRIBNER

SCRIBNER
1230 Avenue of the Americas
New York, NY 10020

The names, characteristics, and situations of some of the individuals
in this book have been changed.

DESIGNED BY ERICH HOBBING

Set in Bembo

Manufactured in the United States of America

1   3   5   7   9   10   8   6   4   2

Library of Congress Cataloging-in-Publication Data
Mathiasen, Patrick.
An ocean of time : Alzheimer's : tales of hope and forgetting / Patrick Mathiasen.
p.   cm.
Includes index.
1. Alzheimer's disease—Popular works. I. Title.
RC523.2.M38   1997
616.8'31—dc21   96-29679
CIP

ISBN 0-684-82252-0

For Jenner

Acknowledgments

I would like to thank my patients and their families for their help in writing *An Ocean of Time*. They gave me the title for the work, all of the stories that appear here, and much, much more. I have changed their names and many of the details of their lives in order to protect their identities. But I hope that their spirit and courage come through to the reader, as they did to me in the course of my work with each of them. They have given me far more than I can ever return, and I am in their debt.

I have been fortunate to have had the opportunity to work with Janis Vallely, who went far beyond the role of literary agent to provide me with the counsel and insight I needed to complete this book. She had confidence that I could do it, and she somehow helped me to believe that I could, even when I wasn't so sure.

Jane Rosenman was my editor at Scribner. Jane had the vision and the creativity to help me shape my encounters with my patients into a coherent whole. Her skill in arranging my words and tales, pulling out the pieces that did not fit and leaving the ones that did, was something that ultimately made this a far better book than I could ever have produced on my own.

I would also like to thank Jane's assistant at Scribner, Jill

Feldman. Jill fielded my endless questions and helped me to get my work in on time, or nearly on time.

I would like to acknowledge all of the other talented people at Scribner who helped me to put this book together. Collectively, they placed an emphasis on the quality of the work which, I hope, will help me to reach out to the sufferers of Alzheimer's disease and their families.

Several of my colleagues provided me with insights for this book. One who stands out is Victor Erlich, M.D., a neurologist at Northwest Hospital in Seattle. Victor read my manuscript and offered me his observations in much the same way that he consults on my patients when I call him—with intellectual passion and sensitivity.

Another person who took the time to review this book is Murray Raskind, M.D. Murray is a professor of psychiatry at the University of Washington in Seattle. He was and continues to be my teacher in the best sense of the word. He is a fine and creative physician, and I cannot thank him enough.

I have discussed the ideas for *An Ocean of Time* with many of the people with whom I work at Northwest Hospital. MaryRose Abejero has been indispensable with her help in typing and printing parts of the manuscript and sending it off on time. Linda Crome has been there for me to bounce around ideas, as have many of the others at the hospital—Bev, Birgitta, Carol, Terrea, Maureen, Tracy, Debbie, Steve, Robin, Amy, and all of the rest, too many to name here. My thanks to all of them.

This brings me to Jenner. She is a part of every word and chapter here. She allowed me the hours of space in the evenings and weekends and early mornings to write this book while I carried on a full-time practice. And she did far more than this. She touched every part of this book with her sure eye and her sense of beauty.

Contents

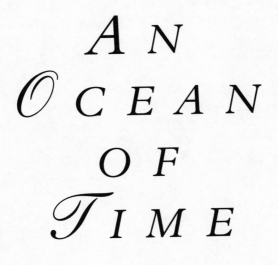

A Ray of Light

Who has not been touched, in some way, at some level, by Alzheimer's disease? It frightens us, pulls at our humanity, makes us want to walk the other way when we encounter it. But there is far more to it than this. There is hope and humor and a chance to gain new insight into the nature of our relationships with one another.

My patients tell this story, beginning with the earliest signs of the disease and passing through its stages right up to the end. And along the way, the uncertainty of the diagnosis arises, popping up like a surprise over and over again.

These are the clinical tales that, pulled together, make up the picture of Alzheimer's disease. But the image is blurred and hard to make out, much like the disease itself. It is like entering waters where a fog obscures everything more than a few feet in front of our faces, and rain whips frantically at our eyes and hands. Just up ahead, so close we can see the light like a dim beacon, the fog lifts and the sun shines through.

In medical training, the art of listening to the patient has fallen away, as if dropped off a towering ledge. It has been slowly replaced by the technology of MRIs and CTs, PET scans and SPECT scans, LPs and EEGs, and all of the rest of the alphabet soup of medicine that takes the place of what was originally there—the patient and the doctor sitting in a quiet room, talking with each other.

We have paid a price for this. We have stripped away the drama of the interplay between patient and doctor. The most important thing that I can do is listen. It *sounds* easy—it even *seems* easy at times. But it's not.

Listening goes against the grain of our culture, where people do not learn to listen to one another. They learn to look inward and also outward into the world and the things that exist within it. But they do not learn to look into the spaces that the people around them inhabit.

The most important tool that I carry into meetings with my patients and their families is my ability to hear what these people are trying to tell me, to separate out the meaning of their lives, and to help them to see this meaning.

This involves more than hearing the content of their words. I listen to the tone in their words, the emphasis that they place on one syllable over another, the way they shift in a chair, the way their eyebrows move as they speak. To convince my patients that I am interested in what they have to tell me, I have to be genuinely interested in their lives.

As medical students, most doctors start out as very good listeners. They are just entering their chosen profession, and they feel privileged to be able to sit down and hear what people will tell them. They communicate this to their patients, who feel it and open up and tell them all manner of things.

But eventually, our training hampers all of this with its daily demands of studies and lab results and one more patient to see in the exam room, and the pressure of too little time spreads out like a pillow that slowly, slowly, slowly smothers our ability to listen to other human beings.

Until finally, we become physicians who rush into the

exam room with a perfunctory "Hello," flip through a chart, and then exit the room in a few minutes after telling our patients what they need to do. And our patients are left with the feeling that their doctors could carry right on with what they are doing, whether or not we were sitting in the room with them.

Psychiatry lends a special irony to all of this. More than any of the other specialties of medicine, psychiatry bases its understanding of the patient on the ability of its practitioners to listen carefully. To become good at what I do, I have had to discard years of training and force myself to sit still and hear my patients out.

No one taught me how to do this. I was taught to distinguish between depression and a failing memory, between psychotic states caused by reactions to drugs and those related to schizophrenia, between Alzheimer's disease and strokes. But no one prepared me to sit quietly in a small room and listen carefully to the person sitting across from me.

This can be exhausting, boring, fascinating, shocking. It can roll all of these sensations together, sometimes in a single session with a patient. I remember an old woman I saw in my first year of training as a psychiatry resident. She had come in to talk to me about her feelings of emptiness and boredom. And somehow, she passed these feelings on to me.

Mavis was slender, in her seventies, with high cheekbones and a long, thin nose. Her voice was soft and low, with a rasping sound to it, and it rose and fell in a singsong rhythm in the space of my office as she talked about a drab gray life devoid of friends and family. I nodded my head up and down as I listened to her words, up and down, until the words and the rhythm acquired a force of their own, and my vision blurred.

In our fourth appointment—it's odd I remember it so clearly—about halfway through the session, I nodded my head forward, eyes closed, and felt a sense of comfort, like floating down through warm water. It enfolded me and I struggled to force my eyes back open as I leaned forward in my chair.

When I finally opened my eyes, I looked up to see Mavis peering at me from behind her thin nose. There were tears in her eyes, and as I scrambled to pull myself up in my chair, I thought she was crying because her therapist's attention had lapsed.

"I'm sorry—" I started to say.

But Mavis raised her long, slim finger and pressed it over her lips, gesturing for me to be quiet. "It's all right," she said. "I understand. Finally, I understand."

My concentration had faltered for only a few seconds. But during that time, the old woman told me, she had continued talking until she arrived at an insight into the nature of a recurrent dream that had troubled her for years. It was a dream from Mavis's childhood, and in it, her mother stood in the kitchen smoking cigarettes, one after another, while Mavis played on the floor. The dream had become more and more frequent as our therapy sessions progressed.

Now she understood the dream. It was a memory of pain, and at first she couldn't locate where the pain was coming from. But then in our therapy session it leaped out at her, and suddenly she knew: It was a dream of her mother's abuse. The thoughts and images had all mixed together in her unconscious, and they surfaced in the image of her mother's face, huge and ringed with smoke, floating above her childhood.

And now it came back to Mavis. She felt the hot pain, and she remembered how her mother would burn her with the brightly lit ends of her cigarettes—on her arms, her legs, sometimes her back. The memory was horrifying for Mavis.

Mavis's mother had died the year before, at the age of ninety-five. Her death had been strangely liberating for Mavis, although she wasn't sure why. Now it made sense to her. Her mother had affected her entire life. Because of the torture and abuse she had inflicted on Mavis, it had been difficult for her to establish intimate relationships with anyone—men or women. Now her death had given Mavis a release, a release and a permission to pursue help in the confines of psychotherapy—something she had never done before.

Mavis gave me more credit than I deserved for allowing her to explore her painful memories. She thanked me for helping her to see what had happened to her in a quiet suburban kitchen decades ago. She thanked me for allowing her to talk about it. And she thanked me for listening to her story.

This is what listening to my patients is like for me. Long minutes and hours filled with the routine, the talk sometimes descending into the mundane details of life.

But always, floating just beneath the surface like long, gray-skinned creatures, swim the ghosts of our present and past—ready to break up through the still water if only the wind is calm and there is someone there ready to listen.

I spend about two thirds of my time working with people whom the rest of my colleagues would, if they are honest, like to avoid. These are the depressed, the forgetful, the angry, the suicidal—and, yes, psychotic patients whom most physicians cannot get away from fast enough.

In the course of my days, I spend several hours each morning walking through an inpatient psychiatric unit at Northwest Hospital that treats some of the most disturbed and troubled older people in the city of Seattle. The patients come from all over: nursing homes and retirement centers, houses and apartments, and the homes of their distraught adult children. Many of them have Alzheimer's disease, and have come to this unit because of complications of the illness.

I have worked in this field for the past five years, since finishing a fellowship in geriatric psychiatry. And I find it fascinating, far more fascinating than anything else I have encountered in the world of medicine.

Many of my colleagues think there is something a bit wrong with me, I suspect, although they would never say it out loud. They wonder what it is that would make me want to work with this group of aging patients. Medicine is a field that attracts intelligent, talented people who like to have answers come to them at the end of their workdays. Clear and distinct answers. And I have always stood at the edge of this world, trying to fit myself in amid the technology and numbers and science of it all. It was this that attracted me to psychiatry, even as I first trained in an internal medicine residency at Montefiore Medical Center in New York.

During my internship at Montefiore I saw an old Puerto Rican man who had taken a handful of pills in an attempt to die—a suicide attempt. He had survived the overdose, and he was sitting up in his bed when I entered his room the following morning.

I was just sitting down to talk with the old man— Manuel—when the attending physician, who supervised me as an intern, came into the room and motioned me aside. We stood only a few feet from the old man's bed, and in a voice loud enough for the man to hear, my supervisor said, "Get a psych consult, Pat, and let's move him out of here."

It was not a particularly outrageous thing to say in this

busy New York hospital, where I often went without sleep all night in my rush to keep up with the patients I needed to see. But the scene and the words have stuck in my mind down through the years. I wanted to talk with Manuel, to hear what had happened to him that had led him out to the edge of his life.

I wanted to talk with him because I was interested in what had happened. I wanted him to tell me. But there was no time for any of this. He was alive, he had no "medical complications," and so it was time to get a psych consult and move on.

This happens over and over in medicine, until it becomes almost an instinctual response to push emotional pain and suffering off to the side, into a box that we label "psych consult." And after a while, as practitioners of the healing arts, we often become blinded to such pain until we can't see it anymore.

This was hard for me to do, to push and force my patients down into the formulas of medicine. It was like trying to fill a box that was already full. My patients didn't fit, at least not very easily, and after a while I stopped trying to press them into the tight spaces.

I wanted to see what was in the box. And for me, the old held my interest more than the young. This is what I was looking for, I think. A chance to learn about life from those who had gone through a large part of it—from some who sat at the far, ragged ends of their own lives and spun out their stories as their very lives unraveled.

This is where psychiatry came in. Psychiatry gives its practitioners permission to bend the rules of the day-to-day practice of medicine, to accept the fact that there may not be an answer at the end of the day. I liked this very much.

The rest of medicine did not give me this chance to listen.

Patrick Mathiasen, M.D.

It demanded my concentration and attention and knowledge. But it also, in a way, demanded that I not listen, because to listen carefully would slow me down.

When I finished my training in internal medicine, I went on directly into a psychiatry residency at the University of Washington in Seattle—a place at the other end of the earth from New York City. A place with some of the very best training in geriatric psychiatry that can be found anywhere in this country.

Alzheimer's disease spreads like a plague from the Middle Ages, stretching out until it covers its victims in a thick, black cloak of lost memory. It is a very personal illness, and it moves into our lives and changes us. It changes what we think, what we remember, and eventually, who we are.

Two experiences in my life, one in childhood and one early in my medical training, led me toward this work. The first one involved my father, who took me along on visits to see his older sister as her memory failed and Alzheimer's disease swept over her while she was still in her early fifties. The second involved a mentor, a man very much like my father, who taught me about life and continued to teach me even as he struggled with Alzheimer's disease himself.

These experiences touched me in a profound way. They influenced my decision to enter the field of geriatric psychiatry, and they changed the very way I view this illness. Now I see hope and concern—even love—woven into the threads of this thief of memory. I see the black cloak of the disease glimmer and soften, as if rays of light are trying to break through the heavy cloth.

As I begin this book, my mind wanders back to a morning over thirty years ago.

I loved riding in the big Dodge, loved everything about it. The gray-and-white vinyl seats, warmed by the morning sun, pressed through my white shirt and dress pants. The huge steering wheel, the radio with its grease-stained knobs, the bump of the road as we hit the potholes. Everything about the car was an extension of my father: his giant hands around the steering wheel, his shiny black shoe pushing in the clutch as we swung around a corner and started the steep ascent, the smell of smoke from his cigarette. Outside, the houses passed in a line of oak trees and green shutters.

I was seven years old, and it was the summer between the first grade and second. The sun came down between the trees, glaring onto the massive hood of our car. It was after church, and my father and I were going to see his sister—Aunt Anna. "Annana" I called her, because the words ran together in my head until I couldn't separate them. *Annana.* Each time I said it, my father smiled and his hand closed down tight around my shoulder. "That's right!" he said, "Annana."

The Dodge pulled up over the crest of a hill, and I saw the nursing home—THE CARING ARMS. My father pulled into the parking lot and turned off the engine of the Dodge. I followed him up the walk to the doors of the building. Inside, it was cool and dark—like a cave.

A nurse led us down a long, narrow corridor, and the smell of the nursing home rose up around me—a strong, antiseptic odor, the smell of soap and detergent and cleaning sprays covering everything. It burned at my nose and eyes, and I tried not to breathe as I walked along. On either side of the hallway wheelchairs sat like cars parallel parked—some with the bent figures of old men and women resting in them.

The nurse and my father each took one of my hands firmly, and off we went down the corridor. We barely fit in the hallway, walking three abreast. Way up ahead, I could see the hallway open up into a much larger room. After what seemed a long time, we came to the end of the hallway and entered the large room. It was bright, with several tables and a skylight above my head. My father and the nurse held tightly to my hands. Behind me, I could hear the faint sound of a patient calling out from her wheelchair.

Up ahead, beyond a small group of people visiting an old man, my father's sister sat alone in her wheelchair. My father let go of my hand and strode ahead of us across the room, leaving the nurse and me standing in the sunlight that fell from the skylight.

"Anna," he said in his low voice. "Anna."

I pulled free from the nurse and ran across the floor to the table where my father stood with his back to me, talking to his sister. He was leaning down toward her as I came up behind them, and I could just see her curly white hair beyond his shoulders.

"Anna, it's good to see you," I heard him say. His voice dipped lower now, and it had a shaky sound to it, like a hand trembling. I came up on the side of my father and aunt just as he kissed her on the cheek.

My aunt wore her favorite long blue dress, and her hair was done in ringlets of white curls. Her skin was smooth and her nose had the long, soft curve so much like my father's. In fact, she looked like my father more than any of his other sisters. She reached out and patted his arm with the long, thin fingers of her right hand.

"Roy, Roy!" she said, whispering my father's name. "It's so good to see you. I miss you."

My father straightened up and looked over at me. His eyes were watery, with a thin film covering them. "Anna," he said, "I brought someone to see you. Look who's here."

He motioned for me to move in front of him so that my aunt could see me more clearly. He put his hands on my shoulders, and he bent down and whispered in my ear, "Say hello to Anna, Pat."

"Annana!" I said. The words popped out of my mouth, like a piece of candy. I said it again. "Annana!"

The woman sitting in the wheelchair smiled down at me. She was only a few years older than my father, but she looked much older. Her smile was a broad, quick movement, and I saw the flash of her white teeth behind the soft red of her lips. The smile grew wider and wider, and I felt my father's strong fingers press my shoulders down into my collarbone. I looked up into my aunt's eyes. They were wide and clear and a light shade of blue, like water.

"Hello, little boy," she said. "Now, who might you be?"

The sound of the old woman's words fell into my thoughts like a heavy rock. *She doesn't remember me? She doesn't know my name?* "But, Annana," I started to say.

My father's hands tightened on my shoulders. "Anna, it's Patrick," he said. "My son, Patrick."

His voice shook again with the odd tremble. My aunt's eyes grew wider as she looked down at me. I couldn't stop looking into her eyes. Deep down in her eyes, I saw bright spots shining like rays of light. I looked at the bright spots and tried to make out an image. But there was no image.

And I wondered, as only a child can wonder, what the bright light was. It was real, like light passing through water, coming up out of an aunt who couldn't remember my name.

My aunt had Alzheimer's disease. The memory of my

aunt and father has stayed with me down through all of the years. Back then, her problem didn't have a single name. It was called many things: senility, hardening of the arteries, a stroke. It was the disease of forgetting, as my mother called it. And it ran in my father's family. Two of his older brothers had succumbed to the illness, and it was something my mother and father whispered about when they thought they were alone.

I've always wanted to understand this disease, this thief of memory that could rob someone so close to me of the memories of our time together. I think back to my father and our visit to The Caring Arms nursing home, and I can see some of my own fears bound up in these memories.

Alzheimer's disease touches us at our deepest levels. Forgetting. Madness. Dying. Images of nursing homes and wheelchairs filled with the shells of what were once vital human beings now bent forward and gnarled, waiting for the end as their attendants swirl about them, feeding them with spoons, cleaning their bodies, washing and fixing their hair.

All of the time, the incessant buzz of conversation: "Oh, Dolores, you look so nice today. So nice. I love your hair. Was your son in to see you? He's such a nice boy." These are the images. Not all of the story, of course. Only the final chapter. But many of us act on these images. I have had people tell me that if they were diagnosed with Alzheimer's disease, they would like to go quickly, rather than wait for the end. They would like to die.

I have worked around the edges of this illness, and as I have worked, my own images have slowly changed. Now I need to come closer to the center. When I work with someone whose memory has failed, an old person who has this illness we call

Alzheimer's disease, I no longer have the sinking, hopeless sense I once had. I see more than the shell of a body.

I see lives that have unfolded. Children who love their parents. Memories that no longer hold together, but shimmer and float upward from my patients, not in a logical stream, but bumping up against one another like dancers moving across a floor. I don't want to romanticize this illness, which has its share of horror. But I do want to tell you more about it, about the balance between sadness and joy and the uncertainty that exists in the middle of it all.

Susan Pearson brought her mother, Mary, in to see me one day. Mary Pearson had been given the diagnosis of Alzheimer's disease. She had been referred to me by a colleague, and this was the first time we had met. She was a small, frail woman, and she entered pushing a metal walker whose wheels squeaked under her weight on the thin blue carpet of my waiting room.

Mary rumbled slowly into my office, and with some help settled into the padded chair across from me. I studied her face. It was lined with deep creases, almost like leather, and they made her appear a little older than her eighty years.

Mary's daughter leaned forward. "Thank you for seeing us on such short notice, Doctor."

At the sound of her daughter's voice, Mary Pearson's eyes widened, and she broke into a smile as the cool sound of her laughter rang through the room. She stared at a point just above my head. I leaned forward in my chair until my knee touched hers.

"Hello, Mrs. Pearson," I said. "What do you see up there?"

Now the laughter became louder, bursting out of the old woman's mouth until it filled the room like a crowded party.

"Oh, Harold," she said, "it's lovely. So beautiful. But God, do you think we can afford it?"

At this, the old woman looked down at her hands resting in her lap. Her daughter patted her hand, and looked up at me. "She thinks you're her husband, Harold. My father. He died thirty years ago, but when she thinks of him now, it's as if he's still alive. She's remembering the day he proposed to her, and gave her a ring."

"Oh, Harold! It's beautiful. Beautiful. Of course I will. You know I will." The old woman looked at me. In the creases of her lined face I saw the light reflect off tears that gathered at the corners of her eyes. She smiled, and the sound of her laughter rose another decibel in the room.

Susan Pearson took her mother's right hand in her own and pulled it to her. Then Susan looked up at me, and now I saw the tears in her eyes as well. She smiled brightly.

"You see, Doctor," she said, "my mother is lost. It's a happy kind of lost. She moves from one memory to another, and at each memory, it's as if she's right there, existing in that moment, in that time. She believes she is there, and so she relives her life each day."

She paused for a moment. Then her smile grew broader. "My mother is lost in an ocean of time."

Alzheimer's disease is not a single entity. It is many things. And sometimes, it is not at all what it seems. It can be an impostor, a reveler wearing a mask, a mystery. At least, it must have seemed that way to its discoverer.

Dr. Alois Alzheimer is credited with defining the illness in the early 1900s. He observed in his patients the tendency to forget, followed by the slow, inexorable rumble of disease as the mind gradually unraveled like a ball of twine rolling down a steep incline. First the pieces of memory, like strings flying from the center. Then language breaking apart in missed words and phrases, until the sentences turn inside out and drop away. This is what Dr. Alzheimer saw, and he wondered, like all scientists wonder: What could this be? What is causing this assault on the brain? That's how I think of him, trying to solve a great puzzle.

He cut apart the brains of patients who died, and he found the pathologic evidence that, to this day, we still don't understand. Plaques and tangles. The plaques were filled with a protein called amyloid. The tangles were tangles of nerve fibers, neurofibrillary tangles. The words are hard to say. They are much harder to understand.

Somewhere in those plaques and tangles, thought Dr. Alzheimer, lay the answer to the mystery of this disease of forgetting. I imagine him peering down through his microscope into the tangles of nerve fibers, clumped together like a knotted mass of string. What went through his mind?

A century sits between Dr. Alzheimer and his discovery, and many, many theories have grown up like weeds to explain what he saw that day through the lens of his microscope. After all of this time, and all of these theories, we still don't know.

This book explores the mystery of not knowing. It tells the story of Alzheimer's disease through the lives of the patients I have encountered. It illuminates the human face of an illness and brings it out from the shadows of everyday life to a place where we can see its many expressions.

Alzheimer's is a window, a chance to peer into the human condition. This is how I experience it at times—as an opportunity to eavesdrop on the most private moments and thoughts of my patients and their families.

CHAPTER ONE

The Hall
of Perpetual Beds

Alzheimer's disease is not always what it seems. Sometimes, it comes slowly, creeping up behind us like a stranger. Sometimes, it comes over us in a rush, and it is on us before we know it.

In a personal way, each individual tells me his or her own story. People tell me their hopes and fears, their pain, sometimes even their deepest secrets. I become a part of their lives, and they become a part of mine. For a short time, I am given the privilege of hearing them in a way even those closest to them—husbands and wives and lovers—do not. But I must listen. I must listen carefully.

Let me start by telling you about Dr. Paul Merlin. Although he was not my patient in the literal sense, he was my teacher, and seeing his decline changed the course of my professional life. Just as my aunt Annana led me toward the practice of medicine in the pain of her lost memories, Paul Merlin helped me define the nature of my practice.

Paul Merlin was like a father to me. My own father died suddenly, in my first year of medical school. And for all of the years that I knew Paul Merlin, I could never separate the image of my father from that of this bear of a man with the graying ponytail.

Paul Merlin was a psychiatrist, and a great deal of my interest in Alzheimer's disease comes from my association with him; first as an intern, working under his guidance in a New York hospital, much later as a colleague, when I saw Paul Merlin himself drift down into the waters of his own memory. It is this later part I want to tell you about, and the effect it had on me to see this strong man enveloped in the grip of Alzheimer's disease.

I received an invitation to Paul Merlin's retirement in the mail one day, and it startled me that so much time had passed. I had finished my internship several years earlier, and I had not been back east in a very long time. But I had to go to Paul Merlin's send-off.

In many ways, he had changed my view of the practice of medicine. I entered my internship at Montefiore Medical Center with my head crammed full of the details of medicine, overflowing with formulas and theories of pathophysiology and numbers and graphs, all of the facts that I thought I needed to become a physician. Paul Merlin helped me to back away far enough from all of the data to be able to see the importance of my role as a doctor.

He showed me how important it was to treat my patients with respect, to listen carefully to them and attempt to put myself in their position. All of this sounds so obvious, and it should be obvious. But medical school had obscured much of my empathy for my patients, and Paul Merlin was able to bring it back both by his counsel and by the example he provided.

He was scheduled to give a talk in the auditorium of Montefiore Hospital, where I had trained, followed by a reception. When I arrived, the room was already crowded with people, and I slipped into a spot near the back wall. I could barely see Paul Merlin from where I stood, looking over the heads and shoulders of the crowd of people standing in front of me. It was a hot New York summer day, and inside the hospital, the conference room was not air conditioned. Two large ceiling fans spun above the crowd, pushing the hot air back down into the room.

Everyone stared straight ahead, up toward the dais at Dr. Paul Merlin—the "Magician," to all of us who came to know him through the years. It was his insights, his ability to take the most complex of situations and distill out the essence of the problem, that accounted for the nickname. He was truly able to work a kind of magic with the patients and young physicians he came into contact with, helping them all to learn a little bit about themselves in their encounters with one another.

One of the men in front of me leaned to the left a little, and I got a clearer view of Paul Merlin. He was in his early seventies now—but he looked twenty years younger. His hair was thick and full, the brown streaked with long strands of gray that moved over his head like waves. He still wore his hair in a ponytail, and from where I stood, I could see the clean line of his forehead where his hair was pulled tight above immense, bushy white eyebrows. He wore a tweed jacket over his white shirt, and his tie had a broad paisley pattern.

Dr. Merlin leaned toward the microphone and adjusted its height. His round, horn-rimmed glasses sat low on a slim nose. He looked up from the microphone. "Thank you for coming. I'd like to thank all of you . . ." He hesitated, and looked around the room from side to side. "You know, I can't believe how many people are here."

31

Paul Merlin was a psychiatrist who had worked at this hospital for as long as anyone could remember. He had a private practice—a very successful practice, it was said. But he devoted several hours of his time each month to working with interns and residents, supervising their work with the most difficult patients.

As I listened to him talk, his voice—perhaps the gentle cadence of his words—triggered a memory that rose up and passed over me like the wind. It came from a time several years earlier, when I was an intern in my first year of training.

Paul Merlin was laughing when I entered his office that day, ten years ago. He was talking on the phone as he gestured with his hand toward a chair. This was my first time in his office, and I looked around the space. On the walls encircling the room hung masks from all over the world—Africa, New Guinea, the South Pacific—all staring out at me. I felt trapped in a circle of eyes, alone in a clearing.

Paul Merlin slammed the phone down on its cradle. He looked up at me, his smile still in place. He was smoking a long, slender cigarette that he held in a gold cigarette holder. He raised it to his mouth and inhaled the smoke deep into his lungs. "What can I do for you, Patrick?" he asked. "Tell me what happened."

Merlin's office had distracted me for a moment. Now the reason for my visit came back to me, and I felt the awful heaviness like a chipped rock in my spine. There was no way to say it easily. "My patient died," I said.

Paul Merlin nodded. My throat was dry and tight, like a piece of straw. "And there was nothing I could do."

"How did it happen, Patrick?" Dr. Merlin asked. His voice was soft and low. "Tell me how she died."

I don't remember much of what I said after that. My voice shook, and I had a hard time talking. "She took an overdose of Tylenol," I said. "But . . . but . . ."

"But what, Patrick?"

"But she didn't tell anyone, until it was too late."

The old woman was a patient with asthma. We admitted her through the ER, and treated her troubled breathing. At first, she got better. But two days after entering the hospital, she took a turn for the worse. I couldn't understand it. It was only when her blood tests showed that her liver was being destroyed that the question of Tylenol came up.

In high doses, Tylenol attacks the liver, and it can turn it into a mass of flesh that doesn't work anymore. This is what happened to Sandra—my patient. The Tylenol tablets she had swallowed, maybe two hundred of them, encircled her liver and shut it down tight. She had had no idea Tylenol could do that. She had taken the pills impulsively, in a fit of anger and depression on the day before she was hospitalized with her asthma attack.

"Was she lonely, Pat?" Dr. Merlin asked.

"Why did she do it? Why?" I asked. "Her husband died on New Year's Day last year. I guess she was lonely—I don't know. And she told me she was having trouble remembering things."

"What kind of trouble?" Dr. Merlin asked.

And slowly, with his help, I was able to reconstruct the woman's history. She had been frustrated and depressed over her failing memory, deathly afraid she was coming down with the Alzheimer's disease that had claimed her husband's life the year before. But she didn't tell anyone, until it was too late. And then, she only told me with great reluctance and a sense of resignation.

There is an antidote for Tylenol's attack on the liver—a substance called Mucomyst. But it must be given before too much time has passed. Otherwise, the effects of the Tylenol are irreversible. If the old woman had only told us earlier what she had done.

"Were you in the room when she died?" Paul Merlin asked.

I nodded.

I will never forget what Paul Merlin said to me that day. He didn't say everything was all right. He didn't tell me that he understood how I felt. He stared straight at me until I looked up into the bright-green eyes below the bushy, white eyebrows.

"Our patients die sometimes, Patrick," he said in a soft voice. "You are their doctor, and sometimes, despite everything you do, they die. Let go of the idea that you have any control over that." His eyes grew wider. "You are there to help, to comfort, to be with your patients in their most difficult times. And sometimes, you're there to be with them when they die."

I sat in Paul Merlin's office for a long time that afternoon ten years ago. And he sat there with me, without saying another word.

"The Golden Key unlocks the Iron Door!"

The sound of Paul Merlin's voice, dropping down from the lectern and booming out through the room, brought me back to the present. Up in the front of the room, I saw Dr. Merlin holding up something in his right hand. It was too far away, and I couldn't quite make it out.

The expression about the "Iron Door" was the one Paul Merlin always used in his mental-status examinations. It was a test of abstract reasoning, without a right or wrong answer. He would simply ask his patients what the statement meant to them. But why was he asking it now, at his retirement party?

The object in Paul Merlin's right hand flashed under the lights. It was small and gold, and then suddenly, I knew what it was: a key.

Dr. Merlin's voice boomed out through the room again. "In my training, there were many obstacles. But they weren't really obstacles. They were chances. Opportunities. Indeed, doors into the future." He stretched his right hand up toward the ceiling. "They were doors on life. But I had to have the key—yes, the key—to open those goddamn doors."

Behind the microphone, Paul Merlin—the Magician— paused for a moment. His right arm remained extended toward the ceiling as he smiled out at us. Then his voice dropped down until I had to strain to hear it. "When I began my training here, the door to the inpatient unit was a large iron door. And I was given a key to that door by my chief resident." His arm stretched higher, above the lectern. "This is that key! This is the *Golden Key!*"

Paul Merlin laughed. It was more like a giggle than a laugh—the sound leaped out of his mouth and fell away. There was a scattering of nervous laughter in the room. It was mixed in with a few hands clapping together in a round of applause that quickly died out.

There was something wrong. Paul Merlin stared out at the crowd, and the smile fell from his face. He banged his fist down on the wooden podium. *"This is the Golden Key,"* he said. *"The Golden Key unlocks the Iron Door!"*

Paul Merlin turned and walked slowly out of the room, abruptly ending his speech. I watched his long ponytail bob up and down on the back of his coat as he receded from view.

I was startled by Dr. Merlin's behavior. It was the first time I had seen him in years, and his confusion—the references to the "Iron Door"—didn't make any sense to me. There was a reception scheduled after his talk, but I wasn't quite ready for it.

I wandered over to the coffee shop first, and as I entered through the glass double doors I saw Victor Rosen sitting alone at the counter. Victor was a neurologist, one of the best neurologists I had ever worked with. We had done our internship together, and Victor had stayed on in New York. He knew Paul Merlin well.

Victor sat on a stool in the warm air of the coffee shop, sipping on a Coke. He waved to me when I entered, and I squeezed between the two black women who were arguing in Jamaican accents and plopped down on the stool next to him. I started right in, without even an introduction.

"Victor, what's happening with Dr. Merlin?" I asked. "I've never seen him like that before."

"I knew something bad was happening to the Magician for quite a while, Pat," he said. "He couldn't remember his lines, the past year or two. He couldn't remember what people told him. And then his wife died last year."

"I heard about that."

"She must have been covering for him, because once she died, he just looked lost."

"Did you see him?" I asked.

"Yeah." Victor nodded. "The family asked me to see him."

"So, what did you think was going on?" I asked.

"I thought he had an early dementia."

The sound of the word *dementia* was harsh and low—and it reached out to me in the hot air like an epithet. "Really?" I asked.

"It all fit," Victor said. "The trouble with his memory. The language problems. The depression." He cleared his throat. "But I hoped there was something else—something we could treat. I did an LP, then an EEG, a CT with contrast, an MRI. I even thought about Creutzfeldt-Jakob disease (CJD)."

"What?"

"You know, kuru, the slow virus—"

I interrupted him. "I know, I know. But why would—"

"The Magician did some basic research at SUNY—upstate. He did some autopsies on the brains of schizophrenics back in the fifties. Think about it. The time frame was right."

I stared at him. Victor began to gesture with his hands.

"And then," he said, "we picked up some subtle spikes in the temporal horns on his EEG. It fit."

CJD was first thought to be a virus, discovered in Papua New Guinea. It was called kuru at that time. The disease is transmitted from one central nervous system to another, mainly by close contact. Very close, according to some of the early work that suggested cannibals contracted the illness by eating the brains of their victims. Scientists thought that the viral particles dropped down into the stomachs of the victims and entered their bloodstreams—finally to rise up again and settle in their brains.

Once the tiny particles settled in the brain, they could lie dormant for twenty, thirty, even forty years. The person who carried them had no idea they were there, nestled into the gray mass of nerve fibers and cells that make up the brain. The years would pass and pass—until one day, like a fish breaking the surface of the water, the particles spilled out into the brain.

It is now known that these particles are not viruses. They are abnormal proteins—called prions—nonliving substances that sleep deep down in the brain. Its victims don't even know they're there. They can't be killed. If we suspect the existence of the prions, there are some characteristics that can be detected. But only if we suspect it. This is what Victor Rosen was referring to when he talked about the sharp spikes that appeared on the electroencephalogram (EEG) of Paul Merlin's brain. This was a characteristic pattern, found in the regions under the temples—called the temporal horns—of the brain.

CJD was a true "medical student" disease. It was exceedingly rare, and extremely difficult to diagnose. In fact, it could only be diagnosed with certainty at autopsy, and there was no treatment available for the illness.

In this way, it was very much like Alzheimer's disease. People who contracted it usually died a rapid death once the prions became activated and began their long march through the brain, treading through the neurons and over the synapses like an army burning its way through the fields of a foreign land. The prions appear to recruit other proteins, locking on to them and changing their configuration. And then these proteins recruit more proteins, and on and on.

"So, is it CJD?" I asked. "Is that what you think is going on?" Victor shrugged his shoulders. He took a deep breath, and then he told me what he had concluded. The findings on the EEG had been an artifact, and when he repeated the study, the spikes in the temporal horns were gone. The spinal tap was negative as well.

I asked him what the Magnetic Resonance Imaging (MRI) of Paul Merlin's head showed. This was the fine-resolution computerized image of the inside of his brain. Victor Rosen smiled. Dr. Merlin was afraid to go ahead with the examination, he said. And when I asked him why, he told me it was because he was claustrophobic.

An MRI requires a person to lie perfectly still in a small space for a long time—up to forty-five minutes—while the magnetic field passes down over the body, realigning the protons in the flesh. Then the field snaps loose and a computerized image is generated as the protons spin back to their original positions.

It is like taking a snapshot of the inside of the brain. Even better than that. The scanner produces detailed cross-sectional views, as if a knife has cut into the gray matter and laid out slices of it on a glass slide.

You can see the vast curvature of the cerebral cortex, the layer that arches up around the rest of the mass of nerves and fibers that make up the brain. Then, diving down through the mass, the ventricles appear—the spaces of emptiness in the brain where the clear cerebral spinal fluid flows—down, down, down into the cerebellum, basal ganglia, and mammillary bodies, the images popping out like sunken vessels illuminated by klieg lights.

"Did he go through with it?" I asked. "Did he get the MRI?"

"Not without a fight," Victor said. "He finally gave in when his son threatened to carry him up to the scanner. We had to sedate him. You wouldn't believe how much Valium the old man took."

Victor Rosen said they were able to get the Magician down to the radiology suite that held the MRI scanner about half an hour after he took the Valium. He was slurring his words slightly, but he was very much awake. It took three techs and an RN twenty-five minutes to get him loaded into the scanner.

"We could still hear him shouting as the door closed behind

him," Victor said. Then he leaned in close to me. "I was helping him into a chair after the MRI, trying to get him to sit down," he said. "I finally get him to sit back in the chair, and I'm leaning over him and Merlin whispers to me, in a voice so soft I can barely hear it: 'The Golden Key, son! The Golden Key! The *key to life!*' He stares up at me, and then the Valium catches up with him and he passes out cold in his chair."

Victor's laughter rose around me, like water bubbling up to the counter. He shook his head from side to side. "It made no sense," he said. "None at all."

It was dark down in the radiology viewing room, with gray metallic light emanating from the viewboxes out into the air. Victor insisted I come down to look at the results of Dr. Paul Merlin's MRI myself, and now I stood with him behind one of the neuroradiologists who was searching for the film. Everything was gray in the room—the desks, the X-ray machines, the pens, pencils, and pieces of paper.

On the screen in front of us, the MRI rolled into view. Every time I looked at one of these studies, I was amazed. The MRI is an incredible tool. It allows us to reach, with the aid of computers, directly down into the gray matter of the brain, where we can see things as if we were holding them in our hands: tumors, strokes, clumps of veins and arteries.

"What do you see, Pat?" Victor asked.

I squinted up at the screen. The film moved from the top of Merlin's head down through his brain, displaying the images of the cerebral cortex and the open spaces in the brain, the ventricles, in clear sight. I looked from one slice to another, and there, down near the base of the brain in an area called the Circle of Willis where a loop of arteries supply blood to the brain, I saw something that bulged out—a weakening of the wall of an artery, an aneurysm.

It was the only abnormality I could see on the MRI. Aneurysms were not unusual in this part of the brain, and they often had no clinical relevance—unless they ruptured and started to bleed. But this one was very large, and I wondered if it was leaking.

"There," I said, pointing up at the screen.

The index finger of my right hand pushed into the X-ray film. Victor Rosen smiled. The neuroradiologist followed the arch of my finger with his eyes, watching where it landed.

"Good," he said. "He does have an aneurysm there."

Victor Rosen broke in. "It's a good pick-up, Pat. We even had neurosurgery take a look at it, but they didn't think it was a problem. And then we tapped him, and there was no blood."

Some people, over the course of their lives, develop a weakening in the walls of the arteries that course up into their brains. The weak area bulges out from the constant pressure of the blood pumping through it. If the bulge is weak enough, it can leak blood into the brain. And sometimes it can burst, in a catastrophic flood.

"Tapped" referred to a spinal tap. Victor had put a needle into the space surrounding Paul Merlin's spinal cord, and he removed a small amount of cerebral spinal fluid. This was the same fluid that flowed up over his brain and then drained down into the spinal canal in its long circular path. If the aneurysm had been leaking blood up in his brain, the blood would have had to show up in the fluid removed from his spinal canal. But there was no blood.

"Do you see anything else, Patrick?" Victor asked.

I looked from one image to another, back and forth. I wanted to find something. But everything looked normal. "No," I said, "I don't."

Victor Rosen was silent as we walked down the long hallway that connected the radiology department with the rest of the hospital. He walked quickly, and I had to rush to keep up with him.

"So what now?" I asked. "Are you going to do any more of a workup?"

Victor spoke without turning toward me. "Like what?" he asked. "A brain biopsy?"

Only the passage of time can make the diagnosis of Alzheimer's disease. It is one of the ironies of medicine that with all of our technology, no definitive test exists for Alzheimer's disease. There is no blood test, no X-ray, no brain-wave recording that will tell us, with certainty, that a patient has Alzheimer's disease.

If we could put a piece of Paul Merlin's brain on a glass slide and tint it with a special stain, then we could look for the amyloid plaques and the neurofibrillary tangles that characterize the illness. This was the point of Victor Rosen's remark about a brain biopsy. Going into the human brain and removing a piece of tissue is the only certain way to diagnose Alzheimer's disease. But there was far too much risk to doing such a thing.

I felt something hit me in the ribs—hard.

Victor Rosen was jabbing me in the ribs with his elbow. I looked up at him. He was pointing with his right arm, the index finger stretching out at the end of his hand. And there, down at the end of the snow-white hallway, was a figure in the distance bouncing and weaving like a cork bobber on windy water.

I squinted and tried to make out the figure, but I couldn't quite see him. I looked around and realized I was in a little-used wing of Montefiore Medical Center, and down at the end of the hall was one of my favorite parts of the hospital: the Hall of Perpetual Beds. That wasn't the official name for it, but that's what I called it. It was a part of the original hospital, built back in the 1800s, and along the wall the benefactors of the hospital had their names inscribed on bronze plaques shaped like the headboards of beds. Some of the plaques were so old they had turned green with age, and the names carved into them were the strong Jewish names of the families that had lived in this part of the Bronx for generations: Sadie Rosen, Samuel Roth, Naomi Nussbaum.

People who contributed a part of their fortune to the hospital were given a plaque on the wall. The headboards stretched down the hall on one side, the names reading like a Who's Who of the Bronx in its glory days. This was the Hall of Perpetual Beds. It was a quiet, serene place, and as an intern I would come here to relax, to think, to escape the chaos of the hospital.

"It's the Magician, Pat. It's the old man."

Victor and I looked at each other and then, as if by silent agreement, we began walking quickly toward Paul Merlin. As we drew closer to him, I saw that he was sliding back and forth across the hallway. He was moving his legs in long, graceful arches above the tiled floor, with his hands on his hips.

Paul Merlin was wearing the same tweed coat he had worn during his going-away party. He was alone in the deserted hall, and he didn't seem to hear us as we approached. We must have been within about a hundred feet of him when I first heard the sound, low and muffled: *"Eee, eee, eee."*

Paul Merlin's back was to us, and the sound wasn't clear. His ponytail bobbed up and down on his coat.

"Eee, eee, eee."

It was coming from Dr. Merlin, as if emerging out of the

back of his coat. I was within twenty feet of him now, and I stopped to listen.

"Key-γ-γ. Key-γ-γ."

He was saying the word *key* over and over. Victor Rosen walked up to within a few feet of him. He stopped just as the old man spun toward him. I saw a flash of gold in Dr. Merlin's mouth, coming from a capped front tooth.

Then an object in his right hand flashed, and I saw between his thumb and index finger a small golden key. He held it up toward both of us as his smile grew wider.

Both Victor and I stared at Dr. Merlin. Paul Merlin stared right back and spun once more, turning away from us and toward the row of plaques that stretched out above his head in a long line of green and bronze down the wall. Then he held the key up to the plaques, as if to make an offering. *"The Golden Key unlocks the Iron Door!"* he shouted.

The words echoed down the hallway through the empty spaces of white tile and the fading sunlight coming in through the windows. I listened closely until I heard the words return in softened tones.

In front of me, Paul Merlin knelt down before the Hall of Perpetual Beds. And then, everything was silence as he fell into the sea of his lost memories, sinking slowly down, down, down as they washed up over him.

When I saw Paul Merlin kneel before the Hall of Perpetual Beds, I knew that I had to know more about this illness— Alzheimer's disease. I had to know how it could affect people, what it could do, how it acted on the mind. Here was a man I had known and respected, someone who had led me toward my chosen specialty of psychiatry.

And now he knelt in front of me, confused, with his

thoughts in pieces in his head. I wasn't even sure that he had Alzheimer's disease at first, although that seemed more and more likely as the months passed and his memory faded. No other cause was ever discovered.

This is a common illness. There are estimates that it affects over four million people in this country alone. And that is not counting the millions more—friends and family members—who are touched by Alzheimer's disease. The financial costs are in the billions each year. The emotional costs are far greater, and impossible to quantify.

It was this emotional toll that caught my attention and held it.

CHAPTER TWO

An Irish Jig

The door swung open hard, like in a saloon, and I looked up from my desk to see a tall, heavy man standing there. He was so large that at first I didn't see the tiny figure next to him, holding on to the sleeve of his green suit. Then she came into view, her ruddy features frozen in a frown.

Without waiting for an invitation, the man strode into my office, pulling the woman along with him. *"Bob McNamara!"* he said in a loud, booming voice.

I stared at him. He had a wide face, with deep-green eyes set far apart. His skin had a dark, reddish tinge, and it glistened beneath the stubble of beard that was shaved close on his cheeks. The man's face, his whole appearance, radiated self-confidence.

Dr. Bob McNamara—the cardiac surgeon. I reached for his outstretched hand, and felt his fingers squeeze down around my own. The grip went beyond firm, beyond strong, and I felt the pain shoot up the outside of my arm to my elbow.

"Dr. McNamara," I said. "It's a pleasure to meet you." I pulled my hand loose from his. I had to squeeze my fingers out between his knuckles.

"A pleasure to meet *you,* Patrick. That's a fine Irish name, *Patrick.* Are you Irish?"

"No," I said. "I'm Danish."

He frowned at me. "Well, Danish Dr. Patrick, I'd like you to meet my mother, Bridget."

With a sweep of his free right arm he gestured toward the old woman who held tightly to his other sleeve. She, too, frowned at me. I looked from face to face, from the old woman to her son and back again. I could almost feel the span of years, like a palpable thing.

Dr. McNamara's mother had been referred to me by a colleague at the University of Washington, a geriatrician I had worked with in the past. All I knew was that the surgeon was worried about his mother, and that he wanted some help.

I studied Bridget McNamara's face. It was wrinkled, with the same red tinge to the skin, and her ruddy features were a mirror of the son who towered over her. She had a surprisingly slim, upsloping nose that divided her face in a symmetry between her eyes, blue and wide. She stared up at me and snorted. At first, I wasn't sure that I heard it. But then she did it again, a sound like a horse makes in a field: *"Grrrrrumphhhh."*

"Pardon me?" I asked.

"Bobby, what on earth are we doing here?" she asked.

Her son had grown silent. He looked away at the thin stream of light that filtered into my office through a high slit of window.

"Bobby, what is going on here?"

This time, Dr. McNamara looked at her. He was startled by the sound of her words, and his eyes widened. "Mom," he said, "you know why we're here! You know damn well why we are."

The span of time melted between them, and the surgeon's voice became high and shrill like a small boy's voice.

"Bobby, I've told you. I *don't* know why you had to drag me down here to see, to see . . ." She stumbled on the words, and the corners of her mouth turned up in a quick movement that spread to her eyes, pulling up the tip of her nose along with it. She looked like she had just swallowed something sour. ". . . to see a sii-kii-a-trist." She finished the sentence, as if she were spitting out an offending substance.

I started to smile, but something in her expression made me stop. Dr. McNamara was looking away from his mother, up at the light filtering in from the window again. When he looked back at me, he was not smiling.

"Dr. Mathiasen," he began, "this has all been a big misunderstanding. It's just gotten completely out of hand."

I nodded, and the surgeon went on.

"My mother lives at a place called The Lifeline. It's a senior citizens' apartment complex. A good place, too."

Bridget interrupted him. "Unless you like to dance, Bobby. Unless you like to dance. Then, they don't care for us Irish Catholics, do they, Bobby?"

Dr. McNamara's face became a brighter shade of red. "Mom, stop it!" he said. He kicked his right toe into a crack in the floor and looked up at me. "My mother grew up in Ireland. In the country. In her village, she was known for her dancing. She danced at all the parties, all the weddings, and all of the wakes."

"That's right, son. All the wakes. That's what I was doing after John's funeral, when that old fool complained!"

"Pardon me?" I said.

Suddenly, I realized we were all still standing up in my office. Before Bridget had a chance to answer, I spoke again. "Forgive me." I gestured toward the two stuffed chairs in my office. "Please have a seat."

49

Bridget McNamara looked toward the chairs and her nose wrinkled up again in the sour expression. "Thank you," she said reluctantly.

The old woman took the lead, and her son followed after her. She dropped into one of the chairs, with surprising grace. No slow lowering, no tottering movements. She smoothed out the front of her dress with her right hand, and went on. "My brother John died, Doctor. I was just saying good-bye to him in my own way. I had a little whiskey, and I put on some of the music he loved, music we both used to listen to. It was nobody's business. I was listening to the drums and stepping to the sound. That's when that old fool started pounding on my door."

As I listened to her, I thought about the reason she had been referred to me. It really didn't match with what I was seeing. Larry Kahn had asked me to see her as a favor. Larry was an old medical school classmate of mine, an internist who sent me a lot of patients. He said he saw the woman once, at the request of the retirement center where she lived. They had noticed that Bridget McNamara's memory had started to fail.

"Isn't she something, Patrick?" It was Dr. McNamara, interrupting his mother's story of whiskey and music. "Eighty-nine years old, and still out there partying with the best. The whole family is like that. Her brother John, oldest one in the family, died mountain climbing."

"What?"

"Yeah, the one whose funeral she just attended. He slipped and fell, and it took them half a day to recover the body."

"I see."

"Patrick, let me give you a little bit of background on my mother. Do you mind?"

He didn't wait for an answer. "This woman is a rock," he said. He emphasized the word *rock,* and the sound of it boomed through the room as Dr. McNamara's thick right hand fell down across his mother's right knee. "She raised a family of six kids. And every one of them, every single one of them, finished college. Do you know what that means, son?"

He was leaning forward in his chair, and his eyes bulged out.

"That's . . . that's very impressive," I said.

"*Impressive?*" he snorted. "*Impressive?* You're damn right, it's *impressive.* Two of them went to Harvard, two to Yale, one to Columbia, and the black sheep, yours truly, to Penn."

He laughed loudly at his own joke. Too loudly, and now his mother's face turned a darker shade of red. She swatted his hand off of her leg. "Stop it, Bobby. Stop it right now!" she sputtered.

"I made up for it, Dr. Patrick," he said. "I went on to Harvard Med."

Bob McNamara was one of the founding members of the hospital in which I now worked. He was a major force in the community, and his temper tantrums in the operating room had become legend. It was said that he would routinely pick up a surgical tray if it wasn't arranged just the way he wanted it and fling it across the room. I stared at his hands and wondered how he could ever perform surgery with fingers as thick as sausages.

I leaned forward. "Dr. McNamara," I said, "would you mind if I asked your mother a few questions?"

His eyes glittered. "Of course not," he said.

Bridget McNamara looked disgusted as she stared straight into me with her dark-green eyes. "Doctor, I'm sure you're a fine doctor, but I don't really think I need to go through all of this. There are a lot of people out there who need your help, and I don't want to be wasting—"

Her son interrupted. "*Mother,* you promised!" he said, then looked over at me. "They want a letter, Patrick."

He said it as if this explained everything.

"What kind of a letter?" I asked.

"A letter stating that you've seen her and she's fine. That she has no evidence of any problems."

"Who wants the letter?"

"The administrator of The Lifeline. I can't believe it, but they're taking this one incident and blowing it all out of proportion."

I turned back to Bridget McNamara. "Mrs. McNamara," I began, "tell me what happened."

I wasn't sure if she would talk to me about it. But she did, starting with her brother's funeral.

"It was tough to lose John," she said. "He was my big brother, the one I looked up to. I've lost other people, Doctor, lots of them in my life, but this was one of the hardest."

Her eyes widened, and I saw the film of tears.

"One day he was there, out in Boston at the other end of the telephone. Then he was gone." She snapped her fingers together, and the sound shot through my office. "What the hell did he have to go off climbing for, at his age. The damn fool!"

The old woman went on to tell me about her brother's funeral, flying out to the East Coast and seeing all of the relatives she hadn't seen in years. It was a grueling week, and when she returned, she told me, she just wanted to unwind and relax. Having a little whiskey seemed like the most natural thing in the world to do.

"That woman had no business complaining about me,

Doctor," she said. "For God's sake, dancing is good for the soul."

Bridget was dancing to some old Irish folk tunes. She admitted the music may have been a little too loud, but not that loud. She just couldn't understand how someone could object.

"You'd have thought I just killed someone, the way Arlene came pounding on the door."

"Arlene?"

"That's her neighbor's name," Bob McNamara said.

Soon after that, the administrator of The Lifeline paid Bridget a visit. And according to Bridget, they had a pleasant chat. Bridget said she had no idea the woman was going to request that she be evaluated by a doctor, much less a psychiatrist.

I asked Bridget more about her background, her medical history, her marriage. Her husband had been successful in business, and when he died suddenly twenty years ago, he left his wife very well off. She eventually moved from the East Coast to be closer to her son Bob and his family. And after several years of living independently, she made the decision to move into the senior citizens' center.

She liked it there. Liked the location on Queen Anne hill, with its sweeping views of Puget Sound and the mountains. Seattle wasn't a city like Boston was a city, she told me, but she grew fond of it. And most of all at The Lifeline, she liked the card games.

"Card games?" I asked.

"Blackjack," she replied.

Not bridge. Not cribbage. She was a poker player. Seven-card stud—one-eyed jacks are wild. Five-card draw. All played for real money. It was a passion, and The Lifeline was filled with people who loved to play. Once she started talking about it, I couldn't get her to stop. I knew nothing about games of chance, and she took me on a wild ride through the games she played. Finally, I had to interrupt her.

"Excuse me, Mrs. McNamara," I said. "I'm sorry, but I have a few more questions to ask."

She looked startled.

"Oh, Doctor, you shouldn't have got me started on all of that. I'm truly an addict of the games."

I asked her questions to test her memory, and she answered them all. She knew the local history, though she hadn't grown up in Seattle. She knew current events. She knew all of the presidents back to FDR, though she slipped up and couldn't remember Ronald Reagan's name. She described him for me: "You know, that . . . that actor."

Dr. McNamara and I smiled. I asked her what she had for breakfast that day, and she was able to tell me—cereal and orange juice. Her memory seemed as good as mine. She tripped over a few words, just couldn't find them. And there were small lapses in her memory. She forgot one of the three words I asked her to recall five minutes later. But all in all, I found no glaring problems. I was trying to think of some other questions to ask her when her son burst in.

"Well, Patrick, will she dance the jig?" he asked. Dr. McNamara laughed out loud, and slapped himself on the knee. "I guess you don't need to answer that," he continued. "She'll dance, whether you and I like it or not. She'll dance right up to the grave. That she will."

I smiled. In my mind, I could see Bridget McNamara swaying back and forth, wearing a green visored hat pulled low over her eyes as a group of senior citizens watched her from their seats around a card table piled high with green bills and silver coins. I laughed, and the laughter spread out in my office among the three of us. When the laughter died down, Dr. McNamara reached over with his huge right hand and grabbed my knee. His fingers squeezed down around it, tight, until the knuckles on his hand turned white.

"We'll need the letter, son," he said. His eyes shone brightly, and there was a pleading tone to his words. I took in a breath.

"The letter is no problem," I began.

Dr. McNamara's smile widened.

"Of course," I went on, "I can't guarantee your mother won't have any problems in the future."

The smile vanished. Now Bridget McNamara was staring at me as well, and I felt the weight of their combined attention. "I told you this was ridiculous, Bobby," Bridget said. "Let's get out of here!"

But Bob McNamara was the voice of reason. He loosened his grip on my knee. "No, no, Mother." He swatted with his free hand at the air in her direction, and for an instant, he became a defiant child. "What Dr. Patrick here is saying is true. There are no guarantees. But right now, Patrick. What can you say about her right now?"

His hand dropped from my leg, and he sat back in his chair. I took another breath, this time a little deeper. I looked at both of them.

"Of course, I can give you a letter," I said. "I can say that I evaluated Mrs. McNamara today, and that I did not find any emotional or psychological problems."

The old woman snorted and then looked away as I went on.

"I can say, Mrs. McNamara, that you have had a very rich life, and that any of us will be very lucky if we are able to maintain our vitality, our spirit, the way that you have."

Bridget McNamara looked back at me.

Patrick Mathiasen, M.D.

"I can say that, at this time, I don't find evidence of any serious problems with your memory."

"That's all we want, Patrick. That's all we want," Bob McNamara said. "Your honest opinion on her condition. That's all we want."

"I'll dictate the report today, if you like," I said.

"That would be great, son!"

At this, Bridget McNamara leaped to her feet and grabbed her son's hand. "Come on, Bobby," she said. Then, as an afterthought, she looked over at me. "I'm sorry, Doctor," she said. "I really do appreciate your time. It's just, all of this seems so ridiculous to me. There was no reason for any of it."

I stared into her deep-green eyes. Somewhere in her features, I thought I detected an uncertainty—a need for reassurance that she was unable to express. It was subtle, buried in the lines of her face, in the eyes open a little wider than they had been before. But it was there.

Bridget McNamara pulled her son to his feet, and I stood up along with them. I shook both of their hands, thanked them for coming, and ushered them toward the door.

"I'd like to say I look forward to seeing you again, Patrick," Bob McNamara said. "But I don't think there'll be any need."

"I certainly hope not," I replied.

I watched from my office door as they moved away from me, down the long hallway toward the exit. As their figures receded, I felt something cool and wet pass through me, like the wind on a Northwest winter day. The sensation lasted only a few seconds, and then it was gone.

Answers come slowly in medicine at times. They are not always found in the lab report, the X-ray, or even in the individual standing in the doctor's office.

One year later, I received a phone call from Dr. Bob McNamara. At first, I couldn't understand what he was saying, and I thought there was something wrong with my phone.

"Hello," I said.

His words were garbled, as if passing through water. And then finally, I could make out what he was saying.

"She's dancing," he said. "God, my mother is dancing."

But I couldn't make sense of what he was trying to tell me. And so, after several minutes of this, I asked him to bring his mother in to see me.

The next day, at the appointed time, they appeared in my office doorway. It was a replica of the scene I had witnessed a year before. I extended my hand, but Dr. McNamara brushed past it, pulling his mother into the office along with him.

Then Bob McNamara turned to face me, pointing toward his mother. "She won't stop dancing," he said loudly.

Bridget McNamara was smiling as she swayed back and forth under the watchful eye of her son, shifting her weight from one leg to another.

"It's good to see you again, Mrs. McNamara," I said.

"Lovely," she replied. "The music, dear. Isn't it lovely? John loves the music, don't you, John?" She looked up at her son, beaming at him.

"John is dead," her son said. "John is dead! You have got to stop this, Mother."

He turned to me. "Patrick, she's been like this for the past couple of months. It got so bad, they wouldn't let her stay at The Lifeline any longer. So my wife and I moved her in with us. We didn't know what else to do. We thought she'd snap out of it. But she doesn't snap out of it. She stays up all night, dancing around the house."

Bridget McNamara broke free from her son's grasp, sliding her bony arm out between the thick pads of his fingers. She spun around and whirled across my office as her son lunged heavily for her and missed.

She stood by my desk, swaying back and forth to sounds that only she could hear. "Isn't it beautiful, John. So beautiful. Why won't you dance with me?" She paused for an instant, and tilted her head back as if to listen. Then she stared straight at me. "It's good for the soul, John. You know it is."

And with that, she reached out and took hold of my hands, pulling me toward the dance floor that spun wildly through her thoughts.

It took me a long time that afternoon to finally calm down Bridget McNamara. I had to listen through lengthy versions of "Auld Lang Syne" and "Singin' in the Rain." Bridget's repertoire had moved from strictly Irish tunes to ones she had grown up hearing.

I talked to Dr. McNamara for a long time that afternoon. His mother sat silent, fixing us with a bemused smile. He told me that his mother had been fine after my evaluation the previous year. She had gone back to The Lifeline, and he had heard no further complaints until about two months ago. Then, he said, the dancing and singing started.

He didn't know what to make of it at first, and as he told me about it, there was a plaintive tone to his words. Bob McNamara stared straight at me with his dark-green eyes and asked me if I thought this was porphyria.

Porphyria is a problem with the synthesis of hemoglobin in the red blood cells of the body. It is one of the famous "Zebras" in medicine, an unlikely illness that can appear sometimes as a psychiatric problem, like depression or psychoses. It is extremely rare, and the likelihood that it was causing Bridget McNamara's symptoms was remote.

I told him this, and he agreed.

"That's what the hematologist said," he replied.

Bob McNamara had taken his mother to a hematologist, and then to two neurologists—searching for an answer to what was causing her to sing and dance to the tunes ringing through her head, alone in her apartment at The Lifeline senior citizens' center. He asked the neurologists if his mother could be having temporal lobe seizures, but neither one thought so. One had even hooked her up to an electroencephalogram and monitored her brain waves over a twenty-four-hour period, looking for the abnormal electricity coming up from Bridget McNamara's brain like a storm. But it wasn't there.

And on Bob McNamara went, searching for the reason behind Bridget's bizarre behavior. He wondered about transient ischemic attacks (TIAs), about the possibility that his mother might be throwing small blood clots up into her brain. The tiny clots could come from larger clots in the heart itself, or from collections of plaques in the arteries leading up to the brain. They could race up Bridget's arteries into the gray matter of her brain, and the brain could reel for a time—a few hours or more—from the effects of the blood clots.

He finally convinced one of the neurologists, Jake Dunner, to work her up for this possibility. But the ultrasound studies of Bridget's heart and the arteries leading up to her brain were free from any evidence of blood clots—"clean as a whistle," in Bob McNamara's words.

I heard an extremely loud tinkling sound. I looked over at Bridget McNamara. She was standing on top of my upholstered office chair, and the sound was emanating from a stream of liquid that was coursing down her leg out onto the floor.

It took a while to get Bridget back sitting in the chair. Once we did, Dr. McNamara went on with his story. Jake Dunner also did a head CT, but it was normal; there was no evidence of a tumor or stroke. Then Bob insisted that he do an MRI of his mother's head. He insisted. "She could have had a tumor," he said.

An MRI was unlikely to help in finding a tumor, if it didn't show up on the head CT. But Bob McNamara was desperate. He was searching for a cause for his mother's decline. And in his search he had pushed his mother's doctors to perform more tests than they could justify with their clinical judgment. In his words, wrapped around them tight like skin, was a pleading sound. But the MRI did not show a tumor. It did not show any explanation for Bridget's singing and dancing. And this, more than anything else, was what Bob McNamara wanted. "An explanation!" he shouted. "I want an explanation!"

His words careened through the room. I closed my eyes against the sound, and when I opened them, I saw a flash of green on the edge of my vision. I turned my head in time to see Bridget McNamara vanish through the open door of my office, her skirt fluttering like the wings of a bird.

I, too, wanted an explanation. I called The Lifeline, and after getting shunted from one nurse's aide to another, I finally was put in contact with the director of nursing, Ronda.

"Hello," she said. "How may I help you?"

"Hi. This is Dr. Mathiasen," I said. "I've been working with—"

She interrupted me. "—Bridget McNamara."

"Right."

Ronda knew Bridget well. Very well. She described to me, over the next few minutes, what everyone at The Lifeline had known for the past one and a half years. Bridget, the strong little lady from Ireland, was slowly losing her memory, her thoughts, even her words.

It had started well before her son brought her in to see me. In fact, it was the reason for her appearance in my office one year ago.

"It wasn't just the dancing," Ronda said. "It was the forgetting."

"What do you mean?" I asked.

"First, she forgot little things. Where she left her lipstick. What time the bus came. It got worse and worse."

"Did you tell her son?" I asked.

There was a silence on the other end of the line. Then came the reply. "He didn't want to know," she said. "He wanted her to have anything except what she has. He couldn't even say the word."

"What word?"

"You know. *Alzheimer's.*"

I felt the muscles across my abdomen tighten. "How do you know she has Alzheimer's disease?" I asked.

Again, there was a long pause. After what seemed several minutes, she spoke. "Well, isn't it? Isn't it Alzheimer's?"

Again, I heard the pleading tone in her words, much like what I had heard in the voice of Dr. Robert McNamara.

CHAPTER THREE

The Prisoner of War

Alzheimer's disease is not a simple diagnosis to make. Many times, doctors too quickly come to the conclusion that one of their patients has this illness. They want to solve problems, to provide answers for their patients. And in their rush to do this, they sometimes miss other explanations for their elderly patients' forgetfulness and strange behaviors.

I was sitting at my desk when the phone rang. The man on the other end of the line spoke in a low tone, almost a whisper, as he said, "I think I might have hurt somebody, Dr. Mathiasen. I think I might have hurt them."

The patient's name was Norman Brown, and he had been referred to me by Dr. David Quarter, an ophthalmologist at the University of Washington. When I called up David, he had no trouble remembering Mr. Brown.

He told me that Norman had been seen by one of his ophthalmology residents, Al Kubota, about a week earlier. From what David said, it sounded like Norman Brown had been having visual hallucinations. He thought he might have Alzheimer's.

I asked David more about the speculation of Alzheimer's disease. Many things can cause people to hallucinate, and I was curious why he had thought of Alzheimer's. David didn't have a good answer for me, but he felt strongly about the diagnosis. He told me that the patient had seemed very confused, and he was in the right age range—somewhere in his sixties.

David Quarter was an outstanding ophthalmologist, and I never hesitated to refer a patient to him with an eye problem. He was always available, always willing to discuss patients with me on the phone. But David knew very little about psychiatric symptoms. And he readily admitted it.

"See what you think, Pat," he said. "That's why I'm sending him your way."

I thanked him and hung up the phone. And as I did, I thought again about psychiatry's relationship to the rest of medicine. In most of the specialties, a common understanding exists among practitioners. There is a set of ground rules from which they operate, a shared understanding of how patients are treated. They all, in a sense, speak the same language. But this does not extend to psychiatry.

Mental illness is separated out from the rest of the panorama of disease. Pneumonia, diabetes, heart disease, strokes, tumors, and all of the rest are cared for by family practitioners and internists and subspecialists. And, for the most part, these illnesses are handled very well.

But psychiatric disorders are different, because often there just isn't time to deal with the problems effectively. This doesn't mean that these doctors don't care about depression and anxiety and the loss of memory, about family conflicts and alcoholism and violence. Many of them deal with these problems. But for most physicians, there just isn't time in their fifteen or twenty minutes per patient to do it very well.

•   •   •

Norman Brown was sitting in my waiting room reading a magazine on the day of our scheduled meeting.

"Mr. Brown," I said.

He took my hand with a hard grip.

Norman Brown was a short, heavy man in his mid-seventies. He wore black, horn-rimmed glasses with thick lens, so thick that his eyes appeared tiny when I looked through the glass at them. His hair was combed in long black strands up over the bald spot on the top of his head.

But Norman's face was the most interesting thing about him. It was empty—empty of all expression. And where the expression should have been, there was a huge void, like a blackboard erased of words. There was no way to tell what was going on inside, behind the lenses of his glasses.

He took a seat across from me, sitting with his legs tight together and his hands resting on top of his thighs. He stared at the small green table and metal lamp that sat to his left. He didn't take his eyes from the lamp when he started to speak.

"I'm a volunteer at the V.A.," he said. "Ever since I retired, I help the guys out, get 'em cigarettes, help 'em apply for benefits, stuff like that."

Norman Brown was a World War II veteran, and he'd done well after the war with an importing business.

"I love the volunteer job," he said. "It's meant way more to me than any money ever could. A lot of these guys have been in combat—they know what it's like. I feel like I'm helping them out."

I nodded. "That's great," I said.

I waited for Norman to say more. He looked at me, staring straight into my eyes with his jaw pushed out. "It *is* great," he replied.

I waited for what seemed a long time, but Norman

Brown didn't say anything more. I told him that I had talked with Dr. Quarter, and he nodded when I mentioned the name. But he didn't say anything.

And then I leaned forward and asked him if he had been having any difficulty remembering things. He took several seconds to answer, and when he finally spoke, there was no change in his expression; his face remained a large, empty disc.

"It's not so much trouble remembering things," Norman said. "It's more like trouble with some of the memories I been having lately."

In early Alzheimer's disease, people often have trouble remembering things. The problem almost always lies in their short-term memories. They forget where they put an important paper the day before, where they left a key to the garage, or the name of a favorite niece. But these are things we all can forget, so the illness in its early stages can be hard to identify.

Often, it's the patient who has the first inkling that something is wrong. And early in Alzheimer's disease, depression is a common finding. The risk of suicide rises dramatically as the patient realizes something is going wrong with his or her brain.

But what this patient complained of did not sound clearly like Alzheimer's disease. It seemed that Norman was distressed over the *kind* of memories that were coming back to him—not with any difficulty he was having with his memory itself. I needed to know more.

Norman Brown said he had gone to the V.A. hospital for an ophthalmology appointment the week before. He had a cataract in his right eye, and it had been getting worse and worse, to the point where he could barely see out of it. Dr. Quarter had been following it, checking him every three months or so. This was just another of his routine visits.

"Only—I saw a different doctor this time. One I hadn't seen before," he said.

Norman Brown was angry, and the empty disc of his face crumbled from the force of his rage. His expression frightened me, and I pushed back in my chair away from him. For an instant, I thought that he was going to hit me. Then he shouted, and the words hit me like cold water in the face.

"Stop it. Stop it," he said.

I was startled by his words, but then my fear was gone, vanishing as quickly as it had appeared. "Stop what, Mr. Brown?" I asked.

He stared at me, eyes wide open and peeking over the top of his horn-rimmed glasses. He was silent now.

"What's the matter, Mr. Brown? Tell me what's going on," I said. I reached out, by instinct, and touched the top of his knee with my hand. It was as if I'd given him an electric shock. He pulled back from me, lifting his leg and turning at the same time. His leg crashed into the table next to him and the metal lamp wobbled—once, twice—and I lunged for it and missed as it came crashing down across the top of Norman Brown's legs.

He looked down at the lamp now lying in his lap, and the expression of terror slowly disappeared from his face. It vanished as his lips sunk back into a frown and the crinkles around his eyes fell into his cheeks. The look was gone as suddenly as it had come, and where it had been was now the huge, blank emptiness once more.

"I'm . . . very . . . sorry, Doctor," Norman said, speaking slowly. "I, I've been like this all week."

"It's OK," I said. "Just take it easy."

I reached over and lifted the lamp from his legs, setting it back up on the table where it had been. He stared down at my hands with a puzzled look, as if they were things he had never seen before.

"I hope I didn't break anything," he said.

"Don't worry. It'll take more than that to break this lamp," I said.

I laughed, but it was a weak laugh, and it came out flat and dull. There was a long silence as I waited for him to tell me what had happened. The seconds ticked by, five, ten, fifteen. Norman Brown sat still in his chair, his head down, not looking at me as silence filled up the air in the room until it was thick as a fog and I couldn't stand it any longer.

"What happened, Mr. Brown? Could you tell me what happened?" I asked.

His head snapped up and his eyes locked in level with mine. "I guess I better," he said.

Norman Brown had gone to the ophthalmology clinic a few minutes early on the day of his appointment, and he had taken a seat in the waiting room after checking in. The room was full, he said, and there were only a couple of chairs left up against the wall in the back. He sat down next to a huge man in a wheelchair and tried to relax.

The man in the wheelchair was wearing gray bib coveralls and a straw hat. Norman didn't get a good look at his face, but he remembered that there were two small American flags sticking straight up out of the back of the wheelchair— one from each handle. And in the man's lap, resting across the front of his legs, was a big box filled with bags of popcorn.

"He was selling popcorn. Right there in the waiting room—popcorn."

I nodded. "What do you remember next, Mr. Brown? Do you remember what happened next?"

"Yeah. I remember looking over at this guy. I was going to

buy some popcorn from him. In fact, I had my hand in my pocket fishing for the change when the TV came on."

"TV?"

"Yeah. There was a TV hanging from the ceiling, up in the corner of the room. I heard this sound, like static, and I looked and it was on."

"What was on?"

Norman wasn't sure what it was at first; it was blurry, and the screen was a long way away. But then it cleared and he saw the CNN logo come into view, and realized it was a news program. The next thing he saw was a large crosshair sight superimposed over the picture of a tank. Then a voice came on, and in the back of the room he heard the words clearly: "Is the U.S. going to war? Is the U.S. preparing for war?"

The next image on the screen was a fighter jet roaring down a runway in the early-morning dark, rising into the sky. And then more jets, one after another, into the desert darkness. As he talked, Norman Brown's eyes opened wide and his hands started to shake.

I tried to slow him down. "Take your time," I said. "There's no hurry. Just take your time."

But it was too late. His mouth dropped open, into the shape of an O, and he put his hands up in front of his face. He was back where he had been before, off in a place that scared him very badly—way beyond my reach. He curled down in his chair, his hands still in front of him, and then began to whimper in a high-pitched sound that passed through his closed lips.

"Mr. Brown," I said. "Mr. Brown. Listen to me, Mr. Brown."

Norman dropped his hands to his side, on the arms of the chair, and his face came full into view. I saw the veins stand out near his right temple as the sound of his whimpering grew louder in the room.

Post-traumatic stress disorder (PTSD) is a syndrome that was first identified during the Vietnam War. As soldiers began returning home from that conflict, filled with the horrors of what they had seen, we began to see young men troubled by their anger and their dreams of violence.

But PTSD existed in earlier wars as well. It went by different names back then, like *shell shock* and *battle fatigue,* but it was the same phenomenon. And when its victims returned home, there was no treatment waiting for them—only a message to celebrate the end of the war, and to get on with their lives.

Norman Brown had been a soldier in the Pacific theater. He was a part of our population who had seen horror and death on the battlefields of World War II. As a soldier, he had been witness to some of the awful things that men can do to one another. Then Norman went back to his home, married, and raised a family. Thoughts and memories of the war and of his time as a prisoner of the Japanese lay dormant in his mind— pushed way down and hidden until one day, the memories reappeared, unleashed like some macabre jack-in-the-box.

PTSD can appear like this, and its victims often don't understand what is happening to them. The mind's defense, its ability to hold the memories at bay, wavers and then crumbles, and the awful memories, stench, and rot of battle come flooding forth. I believe there are many older veterans out there, men in their seventies or older, who suffer from this syndrome.

They begin to have a hard time concentrating on whatever it is that they are doing. Nightmares of violence roll through their nights, and thoughts of death intrude into their days. But they don't know why. They argue with loved ones, and all too often, they become depressed as they try to hide their feelings and move on with their lives.

PTSD can go undetected in the old. Even worse, its symptoms can be attributed to something else—like Alzheimer's disease. Alzheimer's is the great fear of this population. And it is an explanation many clinicians look to when their patients begin having trouble concentrating, when they can't remember things as clearly, when they stumble over their words.

It took me several minutes to calm Norman Brown, to get his attention and bring him back to my office. When I did, finally, I asked him where he had gone. His answer came quickly: "The war," he said. "I went back to the war."

He told me he had been thinking about it for days, had started thinking about it right after Iraq invaded Kuwait.

At first, it bothered him a little, then it bothered him more and more as he remembered his own experiences. He began to have trouble sleeping, to have nightmares. He became nervous, on edge. His thoughts broke through during the day, but he couldn't talk about it, couldn't tell me what the thoughts were about. He could only tell me that the Persian Gulf conflict brought them up, strong and hard, and they washed over him like waves.

"And then," he said, "the nurse called me in."

Norman Brown heard his name being called in the waiting room, but it sounded like it was coming from far away. He heard it once, twice, and when he heard it the third time, he was able to pull his eyes from the television screen and look toward the sound. There he saw a young nurse with dark hair standing near the front desk, scanning the room.

She was calling him in to be seen by the ophthalmologist. Norman still felt as if he were back in World War II, and the things around him—the people, chairs, and sounds—all seemed distant, as if he were looking at them through a fine screen. He shook his head back and forth as he walked slowly toward the nurse, trying to shake the feeling. But it wouldn't let go.

When he got to the desk, the nurse smiled at him. Then she turned and started to walk around the desk, back toward the exam rooms. Norman stood at the desk and watched her walk away. He didn't move. He felt like he couldn't move— as if his feet were rooted to the floor. The nurse turned back, just before she entered a corridor, looked at him, and motioned with her hand, waving him forward.

"It was like I was lost," he said. "I didn't know what she meant."

The nurse waved two more times, and when Norman didn't move, she shouted to him, "Come on, come on, it's right through here!"

The sound of her voice jarred something, and suddenly the things around him snapped back into focus.

"Everything became real again," he said.

He followed the nurse down a narrow hallway, past several empty rooms, and almost crashed into her when she stopped suddenly at the end of the corridor. She ushered him into a room with a sweep of her arm. "Have a seat, Mr. Brown," she said. "Dr. Kubota will be with you in a few minutes."

The name was strange to him. He was usually seen by Dr. Quarter in the clinic, sometimes along with a resident. But this time, David Quarter was out of town, and Norman was scheduled to be seen by the resident—Al Kubota—alone.

Norman sat down in the tiny room and looked around. In the center of the space sat a large machine called a slit-lamp ophthalmoscope.

The machine was black and shiny, with two stools attached to it, one on either side. It rose from the middle of the cramped space like a sleek weapon, like a *Star Trek* piece of metal. Norman Brown couldn't take his eyes off of it. He had seen it before, had been examined by it many times before. But for some reason it disturbed him this time.

Just then he heard a noise behind him, and he turned toward the door. There, framed in the doorway, stood Dr. Al Kubota. Kubota was a young Japanese resident with a round face and short black hair. He smiled when he saw Norman Brown.

"Hi, Mr. Brown," he said. "I don't think we've met before. I'm Dr. Kubota."

But Norman Brown did not see Al Kubota when he turned toward the door. He did not see a white lab coat, a stethoscope, or a smile. Instead, he saw a Japanese officer standing in front of him with a sword in his hands. A Japanese officer in a World War II uniform.

Norman couldn't remember anything that followed. Everything was gone, wiped clean from his mind as if erased by a giant hand. He remembered turning around and seeing a man in the doorway. And that was it; his thoughts stopped there, like a trail that suddenly ends.

"All I remember is looking at that man," he said. "I just remember starin' at his uniform, and then down at the sword. It was shiny, but rusted in parts. I looked at it and I felt this big rush, like wind blowin' up in my head behind my eyes. I felt hate come up my throat, and I couldn't believe it. I couldn't believe it."

"What couldn't you believe?" I asked.

Norman Brown paused. He reached up and slowly pulled his glasses off, bringing them down over his nose. He blinked twice and squinted at me.

"I couldn't believe," he said, "that I was looking into the face of a man who had tortured my friends."

"Pardon me?"

He kept staring. "I don't expect you to believe this," he said. "But I was a POW in World War II; a prisoner of the Japanese in the Philippines. I saw a lot of horrible things. And one of the things I saw was this sonofabitch—pardon my language—with the sword."

Norman Brown bent his head down until his chin touched his chest. It was only when the top of his head began to bob back and forth, and his breaths became deeper, that I realized he was crying. Between his shaking breaths, he got the words out—"I didn't want to hurt that young doctor," he said. "I didn't want to hurt him."

It took Norman several minutes to compose himself. He finally lifted his head from his chest and looked up at me. When he spoke, he remembered the anger that took hold of him as he looked at the Japanese officer. He remembered things the officer had done—terrible things—and he wanted with all of his strength, wanted with every cell in his body, to kill him.

Norman couldn't recall what had happened in the clinic, but he did remember other things—dreadful things. He relived the filthy prison camp and the men dying. American soldiers who died and were propped up in the pens by their comrades so that the Japanese would be fooled into thinking that they were still alive and count them. Then they would pass out rations for the dead men as well, that their comrades could eat. He remembered how the bodies of these men would sit there till the smell was so bad that he would have to remove them.

"The Japanese had this thing about death, Doc. They would never touch the bodies," he said.

The memories rolled on: the friend who died in his arms as he held him; the awful look on the man's face as he took his last breath; the group of men who tried to escape; how the Japanese made them dig their own graves in the hot sun, and then killed them; and the retarded American soldier the Japanese used for live bayonet practice, stabbing him again and again.

"It wasn't right," he said. "We told them he didn't know any better. It just wasn't right."

None of it was right, and it rolled on through his head as he stared toward the door and saw, in place of the young Asian doctor, a Japanese officer gripping a long, thin sword.

"I wanted to kill him!" he said. "That's all I remember. Lunging for him."

Norman Brown paused and stared down at the floor. He looked at the carpet for a long time before he looked back up. "I would hate to have hurt him, Doctor," he said. "Could you find out? Please. I'd never forgive myself if I hurt an American citizen."

There was a pleading tone to his voice, a high-pitched sound like a cat makes when it wants to come in from the cold. And then he slumped back into the chair, and the sound was gone.

Many practitioners have a tendency to clump all psychiatric disorders into one large bag. Then they close the bag and tie it shut. The problem with this is that it doesn't work. These illnesses—depression, anxiety disorders, PTSD—are real things. They are as real and tangible as any disease. They cannot be ignored.

Norman Brown could attest to this. Try as he might, his memories would not go away. He could not stuff them down into a bag. He had to live with them, and the most important thing I could do for Norman was to help him pull his memories out into the open where he could see them—at least for a brief time.

He was like a child in the darkness, trembling as he woke from a nightmare. He needed to feel the reassuring warmth as his bedside lamp flashed on and his room was illuminated in soft yellow light.

After Norman Brown left my office that day, I picked up the phone and called over to the V.A. hospital. I had the operator page Dr. Al Kubota. Kubota remembered Norman Brown very well.

"Sure," he said. "Strange little guy in a plaid suit."

I winced at the description. This was not the Norman Brown I knew, the man who had withstood more pain than most of us will ever encounter.

"Right," I finally said. "That's him."

Then I asked him what had happened in the clinic that day. He paused for a long time, until I thought we had lost our connection. Then his voice came back on the line. Al Kubota said Norman Brown took one look at him standing in the doorway, and the expression on his face slowly changed. "It was like he'd seen someone come back from the dead," he said. "He looked scared. Really scared."

Norman had dived into a corner of the exam room, away from the ophthalmology resident. He hunched down on the floor with his back to the wall, mumbling something to himself that Al Kubota couldn't quite hear. He had not tried to hurt anyone. Far from it, he had tried to protect himself. He had tried to get away from the man he believed to be the Japanese officer who had tormented him fifty years ago, and who was back to torment him again.

I saw Norman one more time, a few weeks after my first meeting with him. He came in to learn what had happened in the clinic that day with the ophthalmology resident. He had to know; it was on his mind constantly.

"I just don't know what I'd do if I hurt an American citizen," he told me again.

The phrase stuck in my thoughts—*an American citizen.* After all of these decades, Norman Brown still distinguished between us and them, between Americans and the enemy. For him, it was a way of surviving the war.

I let Norman know, as quickly as I could, that he had not hurt anyone that day. "You didn't leap at him, Mr. Brown. In fact, you went the other way. You jumped away from him."

Norman was immensely relieved. It was all he wanted to hear. He had not hurt anyone. And shortly after my last meeting with him, Norman Brown's intense memories of the prisoner-of-war camp began to fade away. In a few weeks, they had vanished completely.

I called up Dr. David Quarter to explain what I had found. He listened politely as I told him that Norman Brown had not shown any evidence of Alzheimer's disease. I went over my diagnosis of PTSD, with its flashbacks and awful memories. And when I had finished, he had only one question. "I appreciate your seeing him, Pat," he said. "Maybe this isn't Alzheimer's, but he does have a psych problem." He paused. "Doesn't he?"

David Quarter was right; Norman Brown did have a

problem that fell into the realm of psychiatry. And understanding the origin of the problem was not so hard, once Norman appeared in my office. Norman had the answer himself—all I had to do was find the right questions to ask him and then listen as he told me what it was that was troubling him.

I was thirty-six years old when I interviewed Norman Brown. He had lived more than twice as long as I had, and he had experienced things that I had not. War. Death. Isolation. It was frightening to listen to these things as he told me his story. Each time he banged his fist down, I winced and held back the urge to reach out and make him stop. Each time he traveled back in time to his horror and relived it, I wanted to get up and walk out the door.

My patients must trust me, if they are to allow their thoughts and feelings to emerge. This is the heart of psychiatry—establishing this bond of trust. And nowhere is it more true than in working with the elderly. Trust opens up the space between patient and doctor, and allows the reality of the patient's experience to fill that space.

If I am able to establish trust, patients like Norman Brown can play out their hopes and fears in front of me. If I can see into the drama of their conflicts, then there is a chance that I can understand my patients and help them to ease their pain. This is the goal not only of psychiatry, but of all of medicine.

CHAPTER FOUR

The Journey

Our memory defines us. It allows us to live our lives with a sense of connection to the people and things that have come before. And when it begins to fail, it is a kind of death, a slow vanishing as the body remains behind like some empty piece of armor.

This is a death of the intellect, and it is a very disturbing death. So much so that those around the patient begin to make compensations. Neighbors check in on the old woman in the apartment above them, making sure she has enough to eat as she becomes more and more reclusive and confused. A father forgets a word, and his son automatically fills it in for him, and when the same father becomes unable to find his way through the streets of the city he has lived in all of his life, the son begins to drive him from place to place.

Why do we do this? It is kindness, I think; but it's more than that. It is hard for us to look at what is happening. Many times I have talked with children who tell me their mother was fine, doing very well in fact, until her husband of fifty years passed away and then, suddenly, she could not find her way around her own home. She began to forget the names, and even the faces, of her beloved grandchildren. She would leave the stove turned on and go out for the day.

Alzheimer's disease creeps up behind us like a patient burglar. This is what happened to the woman whose husband died. He had been helping her, covering up her difficulties, and when he died, she was no longer able to conceal her trouble remembering. What she had lost gradually over the years appeared suddenly to everyone around her.

It is a myth that Alzheimer's disease is a defined condition—a solitary entity that does not waver in its appearance. Many people think of it this way, as a crumbling of the brain in which our memories fall away until there is nothing left but a great vacuum where thoughts had once been. But it is not that simple.

Alzheimer's has many forms. It can appear as a lapse in memory, in judgment, in the ability to recall a word. People may hear voices late in the night, as old acquaintances come back to haunt them. Visions from the past arise in the corners of our minds.

The difficulty is that none of these forms are diagnostic of Alzheimer's disease. There is currently no laboratory test that can pinpoint the illness. Our diagnoses must be based on the history our patients and those close to them give us.

But our diagnoses are not based on chance alone. Many studies have compared the diagnosis of Alzheimer's disease with autopsy results of the brain after the patient has died. These studies show that good clinicians are right a high percentage of the time, up to 90 percent. But not all of the time. There is room for error.

This room opens up a space in my patients' lives, an area where I spend much of my time trying to sort through the words and memories that I hear, trying to arrive at a clear diagnosis. In this space, the parade of illnesses that we call the differential diagnosis exists. These are the diseases that can mimic Alzheimer's disease, that can fool us into thinking that our patients have Alzheimer's when they really have something else.

Why is this important? Alzheimer's is an irreversible illness. All we can do is treat its symptoms, and hope to make our patients as comfortable as possible. But it is different with many of the diseases that masquerade as Alzheimer's. Often they can, in fact, be treated. Depression is a good example of this, as is the severe post-traumatic stress syndrome that drove Norman Brown to distraction.

Then there are strokes and brain tumors, Parkinson's disease, blood clots on the brain, alcohol abuse, thyroid disease, and neurosyphilis. And two of the biggest problems of all: medication side effects and medical illness. All of these things are mixed into the lost thoughts and memories of my patients—sometimes a part of Alzheimer's disease, sometimes not.

CHAPTER FIVE

An Ocean of Time

Mary Pearson appeared one day in my office, along with her daughter Susan. Mary had Alzheimer's disease—it had been diagnosed a few years before her visit to see me. Her husband had passed away three years ago. But he lived on, caught in the flow of her memory, rising to the surface at times to play out the parts of their life together.

This is what happened that day. Mary stood just inside the doorway, in front of her daughter, and looked over my office. Then her eyes locked in on mine, and I felt a pull toward her, a gentle tugging that became stronger and stronger as her blue-green eyes burned down into me and my body wavered in the room—leaning toward her, as if toward the edge of a cliff. Mary's mouth opened and her lips framed the words that dropped out into the room—

"Harold, where have you been?" she asked.

The effect that Alzheimer's disease can have on memory is fascinating. The illness slowly advances, taking more and more of our ability to remember the past—at first the recent past, and much later, the distant past. This is a key point: Alzheimer's disease makes it more and more difficult to remember things that have happened to us in the past few days or weeks. We are able to recall distant events in our lives—our childhood, our parents, our marriages and children.

And as this thief of memory marches on, strange things can happen to our sense of who we are. I have seen my patients become quite suspicious of the people around them, including their loved ones. As they forget things, they begin to explain the lapses in memory by filling them in. The car keys they misplaced were moved. The appointment they forgot really wasn't their fault—it was a mistake on the part of the person they were supposed to meet. The check that was misplaced really wasn't misplaced. It was taken. Who took it?

Many of my patients will come to tell me things are not adding up for them. Their efforts to explain the forgotten moments of their lives are very human attempts to reason out what is happening. The explanations make sense, if you listen closely. They hold together, and they allow them to hang on to their tenuous grasp of reality.

But it is not all darkness. Alzheimer's disease usually affects the part of the brain involved in memory before it begins to affect language and our other higher functions. As a consequence, my patients hold on to their verbal abilities for a long time, and their explanations for what is happening to them can be intriguing.

As the recent memories fade away, people cling to the more and more distant past—to things they know well. This can involve a retreat into the memories of past relationships with brothers and sisters and husbands and wives who are long dead. It can mean a reliving of childhood memories, memories so intense that my patients can see and smell the past as if it were here right in front of them.

I am convinced that this can be a healing process for people with Alzheimer's disease. In a way, I think it is a coping mechanism that we as humans use to ward off the blackness beyond the ledge. I have seen patients move back in time to difficult periods in their lives and try to work through them again and again.

I remember a patient who had been abused by her father. As her memory failed, she went back to an episode—a beating she received from him—and relived it over and over. And I recall another patient, a man who had cheated his business partner forty years earlier, who began to wander through the halls of his home at night talking to his long-dead partner, telling him he was sorry for what he had done.

The healing does not only involve a retreat to painful episodes in the past. It can also be a return to more pleasant times. It can be a refuge from the fear and dread of the moment, a way for people to grasp on to their success and hold tightly with white knuckles to their past.

Mary Pearson was doing this as she relived her husband's marriage proposal in my office. From what her daughter told me, the old woman had had a long and wonderful marriage. She and her husband, Harold, were inseparable, right up to the time of his death.

Was Mary's condition a problem to be treated? Could it even *be* treated? I have seen many well-meaning staff attempt to "orient" patients. They will sit down with people with Alzheimer's disease and patiently explain to them where they are and what time of the day it is, all in an effort to reassure them. A few minutes later, these same patients will believe they are back in their childhood, growing up on the farm.

I think there is wisdom in not challenging these people's sense of reality. Families tell me this over and over, in different ways. As I looked at Mary Pearson and her daughter

Susan, I wondered how I could help them. I wondered if they needed help.

"Harold, you damn fool. How could you afford such a large one?"

Mary Pearson was examining her left hand. She pulled it, along with her daughter's hand, over close to her so she could see it more closely. She bent down. "Harold, I love it. But you spent too much money. How can we afford it?"

Her voice rose to a high pitch, and the question hung in the room like tinsel. Susan Pearson pulled back on her own hand, until she wriggled it free from her mother's hand. Now the old woman held her left hand up in front of her face and gazed at her bare fingers. "Beautiful. Just beautiful."

Mary Pearson reached out and took hold of my hands, one in each of hers. She stood up, and the quick movement startled me. "Up. Up," she said. "Stand up and look at me."

"Mother, don't do that," her daughter said.

I interrupted her. "It's OK," I said. "Let her go on."

Mary Pearson pulled on my hands, tugging gently. I rose to my feet, pulled by some force beyond the strength that the old woman carried in her arms. Her hands tightened down around my own as she stared up at me. Her face beamed and her skin almost shimmered in the brightly lit room. In that moment, Mary Pearson's face took on the look of a much younger woman as she leaned up toward me.

"Yes!" she said. "Yes. Yes. We must be married before you go off to that damned war."

I heard a gasp behind me. "My God, Mother, is that what happened? Is that how it happened?" I turned around, and I saw Susan Pearson staring at her mother.

"Is that what happened?" she asked again.

But her mother's gaze did not waver. She continued to look up at me. "We will have the wedding at Saint Anne's. And Father Griffey can perform the ceremony."

Susan Pearson began to cry. She bent forward, and her body shook slightly as the tears came forth. Finally, between her sobs, she was able to get a few words out. "Doctor," she said, "my mother never told me this before. She never told me that she married Dad before he went off to Europe." She took a deep breath. "I don't know why, Dr. Mathiasen, but what happened—it makes a difference to me. A big difference."

I looked back at Mary Pearson. She continued to stare into my eyes. She was waiting. Waiting for my answer.

Alzheimer's disease is not only about pain and frustration and anger. There is more than this. There is also a redemption that exists at the heart of the illness.

Mary Pearson's daughter recognized this. Susan discovered that if she listened closely to what her mother said and watched how she acted, she could learn things about herself that she had never known before.

Susan Pearson was asking me good questions. Why do some people with Alzheimer's disease have pleasant memories and visions, while others have terrifying experiences? Are there factors in the personalities of those with Alzheimer's that can predict their reactions to the illness?

We know that the neurotransmitter acetylcholine is depleted throughout the brain in Alzheimer's disease. In fact, one of the treatments for the illness is to give a medication—tacrine—which increases these levels of acetylcholine. And it has been found to indeed improve people's memory early on, to slow the progression of the disease for a time, to put a brake on the slide toward forgetting.

We know even less about the effect that people's personalities have as they encounter Alzheimer's disease. From my experience with patients, those individuals who have been active, creative people, with strong relationships within their families and circle of friends, have done much better in their struggles. It doesn't seem to matter how rapidly the illness advances—they seem to have more support and resources to handle it.

But these are only observations, not well-defined studies. It is hard to pin things down in the realm of medicine, and Alzheimer's disease is perhaps more difficult to capture in our grasp of understanding, because of all the influence that hard-to-define factors like personality traits can have upon it.

Many, many questions have not been examined. In our rush to understand this illness, we have focused on the technological, and often, in our efforts to produce an image of the illness, we miss the most obvious image of all—the one sitting in front of us in the form of our patients and their loved ones.

Susan Pearson enjoyed her mother's memories. She did not want her to be in pain, of course, but she found that much of her mother's past had suddenly been opened up to her. Alzheimer's disease was pulling Susan closer and closer to her mother, even as the illness spread out through Mary Pearson's life.

Mary Pearson continued to stare at me in my office, and I looked down deeply into her eyes. In them, I saw a glimmer, a bright spot that shone up from somewhere inside of her. The light was constant, not exactly bright or dull. I could not help staring at it. It was very much like the light I had seen radiating up out of my aunt those many years ago.

Mary's hands tightened harder and harder around my fingers until I looked down, away from the light in her eyes, and saw the large knuckles of her hands turn pale. She squeezed and squeezed, and her hands began to tremble.

"Don't hurt the doctor," Susan said.

But Mary didn't look away from my face. "Look at me, Harold," she said. "Look at me."

It was a command, and in her words was a force that became almost palpable in the room. I looked back at her face, back down into her eyes, and now I could see the light shine brighter and brighter, like fire.

"Let's go now, Harold. Right now! You know I want this child I'm carrying. I want to have the child." Mary paused, as if listening. "I have to have the child, Harold. I have to. We'll call her Susan, after your mother. I've always loved that name."

She stopped again, all of the time staring into my eyes. Then her head slowly nodded up and down, up and down. "Harold, I *know* it's a girl. I *know* it is. I can't tell you how I know, but I do."

Susan Pearson shrieked, and the sound echoed through my office. I turned toward her just as she covered her mouth with her hand. There were tears in her eyes.

Mary Pearson looked over at her daughter, still holding my hands. Now, suddenly, Mary is back in the present, rising up into the room from the depths of her memory. "Susan, how could I tell you?" she asks. "How could I? But now you're old enough to know. You are the reason Harold and I married when we did."

The old woman released her grip on my hands and turned toward her daughter, all in one motion. In an instant, they embraced, locking their arms around each other and pulling together as the sound of their tears mixed in with another sound—the sound of their laughter. They stood in the middle of my office, their bodies rocking back and forth as if they were one.

Susan Pearson brought her mother back a few times to see me after our first meeting. I think she did it more out of a sense of obligation than anything else. They really didn't need to come back.

My role in all of this was to listen, to provide a place for Mary and Susan to explore their lives together. There was nothing for me to say, really. No profound insights. No therapeutic breakthroughs. What Susan wanted, and I came to feel more and more what her mother, Mary, wanted, was a safe place to explore the past together.

Mary Pearson would not retain her lucid moments forever. She was passing down into her memory, sinking through what her daughter called her "ocean of time," and Susan knew that she needed to listen carefully and enjoy the time she had left with her mother. This is what she focused on.

Susan had discovered that it was better to accept Mary's thoughts and memories as they came out, rather than challenge them. In the process, she discovered things about herself and her origins that she had never dreamed possible before.

Alzheimer's disease is like this. It is not simply a sentence of doom. There is also a redemption that can be found among the confusion and wandering thoughts of my patients.

CHAPTER SIX

A Voice
from the Beyond

Some illnesses don't appear at all like Alzheimer's disease, but keep the disease of forgetting hidden in among their symptoms like a bird sitting high in the branches of a tree. Parkinson's disease is like this.

Parkinson's disease attacks our ability to walk, shortening our steps until it becomes harder and harder to move through the course of our days. We think of it this way, affecting our strength and coordination. We don't usually think of it affecting our thoughts. But hidden deep in the illness is the power to slow our memory, to make us forget, at times even to cause us to hear voices that no one else can hear.

There is a relationship between Parkinson's disease (P.D.) and Alzheimer's disease (A.D.). Patients with P.D. can contract A.D., or an illness similar to A.D. which affects their memory. And 25 percent of those with A.D. also have P.D. at autopsy. Parkinson's disease can rob us of our ability to reason in much the same way that Alzheimer's disease does. Olive Texas was a good example of this. Olive had Parkinson's. She was referred to me by her neurologist, Arthur Friedman, who told me that she had started to act strangely and to hallucinate.

Olive had started to hear voices, Arthur said, and he wondered if a primary psychiatric disorder was being caused from the stress of her Parkinson's disease. He thought she might have an underlying psychotic illness. I remembered what he said: "This can't be organic, Pat. It has to be functional. I mean, I can't explain it by her Parkinson's, and she's on too low a dose of Sinemet to cause the hallucinations."

Arthur thought that her symptoms were coming up from an underlying major depression, and he wondered if the auditory hallucinations were a part of this depression.

Parkinson's disease attacks the substantia nigra (S.N.) in the brain. The S.N. have nerve fibers that project up to a part of the brain called the basal ganglia (B.G.), which is involved in the control of our movements. Two neurotransmitters must exist in a tenuous balance in this region of the brain—like a playground seesaw—in order for us to carry on with walking, running, reaching for things, and all of the other movements we make during our days. In Parkinson's disease, the balance is tipped.

The two neurotransmitters we are talking about are called dopamine and acetylcholine. If one overpowers the other, strange things happen to our movements. In Huntington's chorea, the dopamine overwhelms the acetylcholine and people move in writhing, undulating ways. The control of their muscles is lost, and they begin to swing and sway like a suspension bridge in an earthquake. Parkinson's disease is the very opposite.

In Parkinson's, everything tightens up and pulls in toward the body like a miser. The cells in the S.N. die, withdrawing dopamine from the B.G., and the acetylcholine rises up and runs unopposed through the brain. The result is a tightening down, a shortening, a restriction of movements that robs patients of their grace and style.

Their muscles move in lock-step, in a jerking fashion like the ratchet of a wrench, and eventually, the wrench tightens down around their face as well and they lose all expression, as if drained of their emotions.

The main treatment for Parkinson's disease is a substance called levodopa, the active ingredient in the medication Sinemet. Oliver Sacks wrote about this drug in his wonderful book *Awakenings.* He described a ward filled with a special group of patients with Parkinson's disease they had contracted from the 1919 influenza epidemic. They were the victims of a virus that attacked the substantia nigra and basal ganglia of their brains. Sacks showed how this amazing medicine could increase the levels of dopamine in their brains, and level out the neurotransmitters so that his patients could rise as if from the grave and walk.

Olive Texas had been treated with Sinemet by Arthur Friedman, and it had helped her to continue walking even as her Parkinson's disease advanced. But it had done something else as well.

"What the hell am I doing here?"

The words echoed through the room, bouncing from one wall to another as Olive Texas slammed her fist down on her metal walker. Olive stood between her two sons, John and Larry Texas. John reached out toward her right arm, catching her fist in his. He held on tight as his mother tried to pull free.

Beside Olive, her other son, Larry, looked on silently as his mother's thrashing slowly subsided—finally coming to a halt. I could barely make out her next words. "Barnard?" she asked. Her voice was quiet now. She cocked her head to the left, as if listening for something. "Barnard, I don't want to stay here. Don't make me stay here."

She leaned her head farther to the left, and her brows tightened together as if she were straining to hear something. Now Larry leaned forward and touched his mother lightly on the arm. "Mom," he said, "Mom, take it easy. Dad's not here right now."

Larry looked up at me. When he spoke, it was in a soft, low voice. "She thinks my father's dead, Doctor," he said. "He's not. He's in better health than you or me. In fact, he's sitting at home right now. But she's convinced he's gone. She's been like this for weeks."

After we got Olive Texas settled in her room, I left the nurse with her and went back out to see her sons. They were both eager to talk, and they both started at once.

"Doctor, what do you—" Larry started.

John broke in. "Is it from the medicine, do you—"

They both stopped and looked at me as I held up my hand.

"Take it easy," I said. "She's in a good place. Just slow down."

They both stared at me.

"John," I said, "when did she begin to believe that your father had died?"

John looked over at his brother, Larry, who nodded his head. "It all started around the time Dr. Friedman started treating Mom with this drug—Sinemet."

John said that at first his mother did well on the Sinemet. Her ability to get around improved as her limbs loosened up and she was able to walk through the house from the kitchen to the living room again. He was amazed. But then, odd things started to happen.

Larry jumped into the conversation here. He said his mother began to point at spots on the floor and ask her husband to get rid of the spider she saw running there. But no one else could see the spider. Then she saw other things— first small animals, then an old cocker spaniel that had died years ago. Larry said no one could convince his mother that these things weren't there.

"But that wasn't the worst of it," Larry said. "The worst was when she began to hear the voices."

Olive Texas began to hear voices at night, soft and low sounds that she couldn't make out. Then the voices spread to the daytime, and became louder and louder. "Until they finally became one voice," John said. "My father's voice."

Olive Texas suffered side effects from the medication Sinemet. I believed that the same drug that had allowed her to move more freely had also brought on her hallucinations and strange beliefs.

The dopamine levels had increased in the spaces between the neurons of her brain. The levels had climbed and climbed as the Sinemet worked its magic, until the dopamine flooded through her brain and she began to walk and smile again. But along with this came hallucinations.

We know that dopamine is associated with psychosis. There are several dopamine receptors in the brain, many of them in the limbic system. Schizophrenics have either too much dopamine or dopamine that doesn't work right. Their hallucinations seem to be caused by this dopamine, and the major treatment is to give medication that blocks the effects of the dopamine at the neurotransmitter level. Medicines like Haldol, Thorazine, or Mellaril.

In Olive Texas's case, the Sinemet had caused the dopamine levels to rise, offsetting the loss of this transmitter in the basal ganglia deep in her brain. The hallucinations and delusions had flowed out into her thoughts, just as her movements began to flow again.

But it wasn't quite so simple. Olive Texas also had a failing memory; there are estimates that 30 percent or more of people with Parkinson's disease develop problems with their memory and thoughts. The difficulties are very similar to those of Alzheimer's disease—in some cases, identical. These unfortunate patients need to be treated for both of their problems: the Alzheimer's and the Parkinson's disease.

Olive's sons told me that she had been diagnosed with Parkinson's disease seven years earlier. But her memory had started to fail only in the past couple of years. They noticed it with small things at first. Olive had been a wonderful cook all of her life, especially fascinated with French and Italian food. But she began to misplace her recipes, to forget the amounts of the ingredients in her favorite dishes. Eventually, she could not remember how to work the oven, and she would sometimes turn it on and leave the house.

The troubles went on. She became lost going to familiar places, couldn't find her way through neighborhoods she had lived in for years. Her sons became more and more alarmed.

Now she was waking in the night confused, wondering where she was and crying out. At first, her husband couldn't make out her words. They were only garbled sounds, the words not even recognizable. But one night they became clear, and he heard something that terrified him: "Barnard, why did you leave me? You *bastard*, why did you die?"

He heard the questions over and over through his nights, and it frightened him and he didn't know what to do. He couldn't believe that Olive, his dear wife, thought he was dead and gone.

How much of Olive's belief that her husband was dead was caused by the Sinemet? How much by advancing Parkinson's disease? How much by the onset of a dementia very much like Alzheimer's disease? What was going on with Olive Texas?

My patients' families, their husbands, wives, and children, often ask me what it means when their loved ones begin to act in strange and bizarre ways. Barnard Texas wanted to know why his wife believed he had died.

I was the psychiatrist, and he wanted an interpretation of the behavior. He wanted me to go beyond the explanation that the neurotransmitters in her brain were malfunctioning, that they were not carrying their messages through the spaces between the nerves in a way that made sense to the brain. And I didn't have a good answer for him.

Maybe there was too much dopamine climbing up over the ramparts of her neurons and infiltrating her thoughts. He could accept this as part of the reason. But he wanted more. He wanted me to help him to come to a place where he could live with the strangeness of it all.

This is the difficult part of my practice. If I am honest with myself and my patients, I have to admit that I don't have answers to all of their questions. Olive Texas had developed the delusional belief that her husband had died, and even though he stood there right in front of her, she clung to the belief. What purpose did it serve for her? She had no history of emotional problems or mental disorders. In fact, she had done well throughout her life. She had managed to marry and raise a family.

So I told her husband that I didn't have a single answer to his question. But I told him that I had some thoughts about what was happening to his wife, and as long as he didn't view them as the *only* answer, they might be helpful. Barnard had some trouble with this approach.

"You mean you don't know?" he asked.

I nodded. "I think your wife loves you very much, and she is afraid of losing you," I said.

Barnard listened intently as I went on. I told him that perhaps his wife's strange belief that he had died was an expression of her greatest fear—her fear of losing him. Woven into the fear was her desperate wish for a closer relationship with Barnard, and it was reflected in his voice echoing through her head, talking to her as he had never talked to her when he was alive. She even said it in so many words: "You never talked loud enough when you were alive."

Barnard Texas looked at me, and his eyes widened. "Are you sure about this?" he asked.

"No," I said, "not completely."

And then I went on. I told Barnard that I believed Olive's wish was a desire to pull closer to him so that she could tell him her thoughts and dreams. It was her wish for a more intimate relationship, and I told Barnard he should feel honored by Olive's attempt.

Barnard Texas smiled at me when I finished. "I'll have to think about that," he said. "I never did listen to her the way I should have."

Olive Texas was in the hospital for over a month. And during that time, I tried everything. We stopped her Sinemet, because the medication seemed to be at least part of her problem. Gradually, Olive stiffened up as the dopamine leached out of the spaces between her nerves and left her body.

It was a slow process, like watching water freeze on a cold, cold morning. Olive moved more slowly, and more slowly still, until she could not move at all and had to be helped from her chair by the aides. Finally, one day she could not even rise with the help of others—she just sat in her wheelchair and stared up at us. This was the trade-off, I thought, the penalty for erasing her belief that her husband had died.

But it was no good! Olive clung tightly to the idea that her husband was dead and gone. She laughed at me when I brought Barnard into the room right in front of her, trying to confront her false belief with the man she had lived with for over forty years.

"You're crazy," she said, slapping her knee with her hand. "Crazy, crazy, crazy, crazy."

Her voice drifted down in intensity, like a rock falling through green water. And then she started to laugh at the sound of the word. "*Crazy,*" she said. "That's not good for a head doctor, is it?"

I started Olive back on the Sinemet, and in a few days, she was out of her wheelchair and walking along the halls of our unit. She continued to stare right through her husband, as if he didn't exist. But at least she was walking.

Next, I tried Olive on a low dose of an old antipsychotic medication, Haldol. She seemed to handle it well at first, and it calmed her down to the point where I could talk with her. Haldol works by blocking the receptors for the transmitter dopamine in the brain. Unfortunately, Haldol can block the benefits of Sinemet as well.

I watched Olive Texas carefully. Things went well for the first few days. She glided through the unit behind her walker, sliding in silence down the carpeted hallways and over the linoleum in the kitchen area. I watched her face—wide open, smiling. And then it struck suddenly.

Olive was standing in the doorway to her room, leaning

down on her walker and staring at the ground. I entered the archway and stopped. "Good morning," I said.

I reached out to touch her on the arm. Just as my fingers pressed against her skin, her head snapped up and a rush of air came roaring out of her lungs like the whine of a race car. I jumped back from the doorway and bumped into someone behind me. It was Liz, one of our unit nurses.

"What's the matter, Pat?" Liz asked.

I looked back toward Olive Texas. She stood straight up above her metal walker, her head pushed back and her neck twisted way to the right. Her eyes rolled back in her head, and all I could see were the white parts. She looked in agony. She looked possessed.

"Liz," I said, "get fifty milligrams of Benadryl, stat."

Liz rushed down the hall toward the nursing station, leaving me to stare at Olive. She continued to arch her head back over her right shoulder, until I was looking at the hair on the back of her skull. I thought of the scene in *The Exorcist* in which the child's head turns completely around on her shoulders. Olive Texas stood stock-still, frozen in place.

She was having an acute dystonic reaction. A sudden stiffening of the muscles in her neck and face, even in her eyes, was causing the frightening grimace I saw etched into her features.

This is an unpredictable side effect of antipsychotic medications. It can happen to any patient given the medication. The balance between acetylcholine and dopamine becomes upset, and along with this there appears to be shifts in the sensitivities of the dopamine and acetylcholine receptors. In the end, the acetylcholine overwhelms the dopamine.

This is only part of the problem, and the mechanism is not completely understood. In some ways, the effect mimics what happens in Parkinson's disease itself, when dopamine levels fall in the brain and moving about becomes more and more difficult. But with a dystonic reaction, the stiffening comes on suddenly, and all at once. The antidote is to balance out the levels between acetylcholine and dopamine. In this case, the acetylcholine overwhelmed the dopamine, and the effect was to freeze Olive Texas's face in a contorted expression of fear.

I had to find something that would counter the effects of the acetylcholine in Olive Texas. This is where Benadryl comes in. Benadryl is a common over-the-counter medication, used to treat allergies and colds. But it is also a strong anticholinergic agent, and when given as a shot into a patient's muscles, it acts to reduce the effects of the acetylcholine in the brain, to enable the dopamine to pull up level with the acetylcholine. The Benadryl helps to lighten the effects of the acetylcholine—it brings it into alignment with the dopamine.

"I've got ahold of her arms, Liz. Go ahead and give her the shot."

Liz pushed the needle into Olive's arm and injected the Benadryl. The effect took a few seconds to take hold. Then Olive's eyes spun forward, and the white vanished as the color of her pupils appeared again. Her face fell back into its soft folds of skin as her eyes opened up and her neck unwound.

Olive frightened me. Her delusion of her husband's death was so powerful, so intense, that I felt pulled into it like a small shaving of metal in the grip of a magnet.

As I watched Olive Texas walk down the long, narrow hallway of our unit, her back receding, she passed several other patients who stood along her path. I thought of what it was

Patrick Mathiasen, M.D.

like to work on a psychiatry unit among some of the most disturbed elderly patients.

I wasn't thinking of "disturbed" in the angry, sad, nervous sense—although many of my patients had those qualities. I was thinking of those who, like Olive, had broken loose from their familiar surroundings and had fallen into a maelstrom of hallucinations and delusions—in a word: into psychosis.

What is it like to work amid the madness of a patient who believes her husband has died when he stands directly in front of her? Or among those who see visions of frightening apparitions who visit their rooms late at night, and scream out even as the nurse turns on the light? Or those who believe, as one of my patients did, that they are prisoners in a federal institution locked up for reasons they don't understand and visited on a daily basis by the warden—their psychiatrist—who will not tell them why they are there or what is going to happen to them next?

I find this place where my patients go a fascinating place, a world unlike the one most of us exist in. Most psychiatrists, if they are honest, will admit to this fascination. We all entered medicine because we wanted to help people. But there is more than that; there is the intellectual interest in disease, and for psychiatrists, the diseases are diseases of the mind. We are interested in the wild extremes of human behavior, as much as or more than in the definition of what is "normal."

My job is to bring people back from these extremes, or if that's not possible, then to help them to come to terms with living on the wild edge of existence. To do this work, I am given permission to enter places most of us cannot go, like a foreign traveler with a special visa.

I walk along through our inpatient unit, with its double rooms spreading out on either side of a narrow hallway.

When the unit is filled with patients, as it often is, the sounds can rise up on each side of the corridor and meet in the middle of the space as I walk along. Some are low-pitched guttural sounds, like growls; others are high-pitched screeches. There are men and women wandering through the hallway, searching for misplaced objects and people and pets, asking where they are and why they are there.

These are people in pain, and we are trying to help them. They are people who have lost their way, and in many cases, pulled their families along with them into the confusion of their wanderings. Many but not all of them have Alzheimer's disease and are experiencing complications of this dread illness. In their pain, they say things that are unexpected, and their statements jar me, force me to think and to see the world in a different way.

This is what I like about working on our hospital unit. It is a difficult place to be at times. But these same qualities afford me the chance to encounter my patients from strange and unusual angles, and these angles force me to see, hear, and understand life in ways that I never dreamed possible. This is a privilege.

Barnard Texas could not accept his wife's belief that he was dead. He just could not accept it.

I did not have a good answer for him. There are no good answers to psychosis. I tried other things. I tried a new medication called Risperdal, an antipsychotic similar to Haldol. It was supposed to be effective for patients who didn't respond to the more traditional medicines. It blocked a different pattern of chemical receptors in the neural spaces, and it was less likely to cause the stiffening that the Haldol had caused with Olive.

Olive tolerated the medication without a problem. Unfortunately, it had no effect on her belief that her husband was dead. And Barnard sat in the background through all of this, peering over my shoulder and watching closely— as closely as he had watched when Olive had her dystonic reaction.

Olive Texas was discharged from our hospital to a nursing home. Barnard didn't want her to go there, but there was really no alternative. She could not take care of herself, with her Parkinson's disease and her failing memory, and Barnard could not help her because, in her mind, he had ceased to exist.

Six months after Olive was discharged, I received a call from the administrator of the nursing home. He asked me if I could do a follow-up visit, to check in on her. He said I would be surprised when I saw her again. I thought that was odd. I couldn't imagine anything about Olive that would surprise me, after her stay on our unit.

I arrived at the nursing home on a Wednesday evening, and stood in front of the door to Olive's room. The door was open, and Olive's room was dark as I entered. I stopped for a minute, to allow my eyes to adjust. The door to the bathroom was closed, and on the far side of the room a slender form sat in a wheelchair by a darkened window. I squinted and walked partway across the room. Then the figure came into focus. It was Olive Texas, sitting all alone, wrapped in a thin cotton shawl.

"Olive!" I called out. "It's nice to see you."

She didn't answer at first, and I wasn't sure if she had heard me. I tried again. "Olive?"

The old woman jumped back in her chair and almost fell out of it. She looked up at me. "My God, Doctor, you nearly scared me to death," she said.

"I'm sorry, Olive," I said.

Olive Texas looked good, even in the darkened room. She had put on some weight, and she carried it well. There was a long pause as we studied each other. Olive spoke first. "I found him," she said.

"Pardon me?"

"I found Barnard. Least, that's what I tell him. I don't know how, Doctor, but I found him." Her voice dropped to a low whisper in the room. "I crossed over," she said.

"Crossed over?"

"To the other side!" she said, then gestured with her right hand, making a fist with the thumb pointed down toward the ground. She grinned. "Death! Death!" she said. "I'm dead, and you can see me only because you're one of those special people that can cross from life over to death. That's why you could see Barnard before, when I couldn't."

Olive stopped and took a deep breath. I saw her chest rise up as air filled her lungs. "It all makes sense to me now," she said.

At that instant, light flooded through the room and I was blinded. I held up my hand to shield my eyes, and a voice boomed out through the room.

"Doctor, where the hell have you been?"

I recognized the voice instantly. It was Barnard Texas. Slowly, he came into focus, standing near the bathroom door with his hand on the light switch to the room. Barnard looked good. He had put on some weight as well, and he looked relaxed. Most amazing, though, was his smile. I had never seen him smile before—the white of his teeth flashed under the fluorescent lights.

"Mr. Texas," I said, "it's good to see you. How are you?"

"How am I?" He repeated the question. "How am I?" His

smile grew broader. "Doctor, this sweet lady here helped me to understand what had happened to me. She helped me to see, to really see, that I was no longer among the living. And then, goddamn, she came over and joined me."

He laughed, and his smile grew wider. "You know, death ain't so bad. You should try it sometime."

CHAPTER SEVEN

The Cuban
Baseball Team

Lawrence McGlynn came into the hospital one day, accompanied by his wife, Karen. Lawrence was chased by the visions that invaded his sleep at night, visions that eventually drove him out to an avenue where headlights filled the darkness of his dreams.

Lawrence McGlynn was seventy-five years old, although he looked at least fifteen years younger. He stood ramrod straight in the interviewing room where I first met with him and his wife.

Together, these two looked like the ideal elderly couple—strong and clear and bright in the confines of the small green room that sat near our inpatient unit. As I looked at them, I hoped that I could age as gracefully. I motioned for them to have a seat at the round table in the center of the room.

I studied Lawrence McGlynn's face as he pulled out a chair and slid smoothly as a cat into it. There were almost no lines on his features—the skin was smooth and tight, and it glistened under the fluorescent light in the room. His brown hair was clipped short, in military fashion, and he was clean-shaven. Lawrence had high cheekbones, and his eyes

107

were a gray-blue color, like gunmetal. They captured my attention. He stared straight at me, without blinking.

Lawrence folded his hands together, one on top of the other, on the table in front of him. His wife reached over, put her hand on top of his, and squeezed. She began the conversation.

"My husband was diagnosed with Alzheimer's disease four years ago, Dr. Mathiasen. He has lived at home since that time, without any problems."

The word *problems* rang through the room, like a challenge. I nodded my head slowly up and down as Mrs. McGlynn went on. "In the last few weeks, Larry has been waking up at night, and he gets up to pace about the house. And then the other night, he ran away."

Lawrence McGlynn took his hand out from under his wife's hand and patted her arm gently. "Honey, don't worry about it," he said. "It's nothing. I got through the army, and the rangers. I can get through this." He turned and looked at me. "I was in the Special Forces, in the Pacific theater. And thank God, I got most of my men through it. But I saw good friends of mine get killed, some of them no more far away than from me to you."

Lawrence McGlynn was an articulate man, almost too well-spoken for a man four years into his Alzheimer's disease. But Alzheimer's could be like this. I have seen many patients with parts of their language well preserved, especially around topics which they felt strongly about. Lawrence was like this.

He pulled his shoulders back and sat up a little straighter in his chair. He tilted his head back a little bit, and thrust his jaw forward until it jutted out toward me over the table.

"Let me tell you what happened the other night in my bedroom. See what you make of it."

Both Karen and Lawrence McGlynn leaned in toward me, and this is what they recounted.

It was cool in their bedroom that night, a November night with the wet dampness of the Northwest hanging in the air. Karen remembered they had pulled one of their large wool comforters out of the closet for the first time that season.

Lawrence heard something—a noise like a scratching sound coming from downstairs. He got up to investigate, and Karen heard him as he padded down the carpeted stairway in his bare feet. She was near sleep, and her husband had been wandering in the night for weeks now. She decided that if he didn't come back in a few minutes, she would get up to check on him.

Lawrence came back to bed much later—maybe an hour or more later. He couldn't recall what he did downstairs, but he knew that he didn't find anything that was making the noise.

"I don't know. Maybe it was a cat," he said.

His wife broke in. "We don't have a cat, Larry."

"Maybe the neighbor's cat," he said.

What happened next was confusing. Lawrence went back to bed and fell asleep almost immediately, from what his wife remembered. But Karen lay awake for a long time, maybe an hour or more. She stared up at the high ceiling in their bedroom, trying to make out the cracks that ran along the painted tiles. She was worried about her husband, and the worry kept her awake.

Karen thought she heard a noise downstairs as well, a scratching sound. But it was faint, and it came just as she was falling off to sleep. That's the last thing she remembered, until her husband's scream awakened her. When she opened her eyes, the first thing she saw was her husband's legs in front of her. She looked up, from his feet up his calves and thighs. And there, towering above her, Lawrence McGlynn stood on top of the bed in his nightclothes—his arms stretched straight out in front of him.

Lawrence picked up the story there. "I don't know how they got in the room," he said. "I just have no idea."

Lawrence McGlynn's mouth dropped open and his eyes squinted out at me. It was a look of fear.

"What did you see, Mr. McGlynn?" I asked.

Now, his mouth began to tremble. "I saw . . ." He paused. "I saw the Cuban baseball team that I played for. But it couldn't be—it was over forty years ago, before Castro."

Karen reached over and squeezed her husband's arm. She smiled at him, and he went on. "But there they were. There they were, at least some of them. Tito and Manny and Edgar. They were standing around the bed, staring at me."

Karen McGlynn told me she saw nothing in the room except her husband standing up on the bed, screaming out in a high-pitched voice, *"Leave me alone! Leave me alone!"*

Lawrence leaped off the bed and ran from the room. He remembered the baseball players, dressed in uniforms from the late 1940s, reaching out at him, trying to stop him as he ran.

"But their hands went right through me, like they weren't even there," he said.

He ran down the stairs of his house and out the front door, screaming into the night like the whistle of a train rolling down the rails. Lawrence couldn't remember where he went or what he did after he left the house. His wife filled in some of the gaps.

"We found him out on Aurora Avenue, in the parking lot of a motel. It wasn't a very good part of Aurora," she said.

Lawrence McGlynn had run out through the night, down past the cars and bars in his bedclothes, not knowing where he was going but heading toward a place he knew from the past. Down past the furtive drug dealers and traffic lights and oncoming traffic, past the hookers and cheap hotels that strung out one after another on this seedy street of lost dreams called Aurora. And something pulled him toward one place among many: *The Last Call Motel.*

That's where Karen and her son found Lawrence, in the early morning several hours after he had run screaming from the house. He was huddled in the parking lot, leaning up against the wheel well of a pickup truck with wheels jacked up and a rifle rack in the back window. When Karen found him, he was rocking back and forth and calling out, "Belinda . . . Belinda, I'm so sorry."

Belinda was the name of his first wife, a woman he rarely talked about from a marriage that had ended in divorce. The Last Call Motel was the place he had stayed when Belinda kicked him out of the house over thirty-five years ago.

Karen had gone there looking for him on a hunch. The motel had been completely rebuilt over the years, but it still carried the same name, and now that name blinked out in red neon, shining through the falling rain of a Northwest night. Below the name, in a softer green neon, the word VACANCY glowed out—with the letter V burned out.

Karen and their son, Brian, pulled Lawrence up to his feet from the gravel of the parking lot. He watched his wife suspiciously as she brushed the rocks and sand from his pajamas. "Don't," Lawrence said. "Don't. I'm safe here. I'm safe here. Don't make me go back."

He kept repeating the words *I'm safe here,* over and over, and it took Karen and Brian a long time to persuade

111

Lawrence to get in the car and ride back to the house with them.

When Karen and Lawrence finished their story, they both leaned back in their chairs, as if by some agreed signal, and looked at me. Karen spoke first.

"Is this Alzheimer's disease, Doctor? Do you see this in Alzheimer's?"

It is crucial in my work with my patients and their families to be as honest as I can be. So I looked at both of them and tried to choose my words carefully.

"I see a lot of different things in Alzheimer's disease," I said. "But this is a little"—I struggled for the right word—"a little unusual," I said, completing the sentence.

Karen nodded, and her tightly curled brown hair fluttered on her head. Lawrence continued to watch me—his expression didn't change. They waited for me to say more.

I smiled and took a breath. "The hallucinations you had, Mr. McGlynn, of the baseball players—that isn't really classic for the disease."

Karen and Lawrence continued to watch me, and I regretted using the word *classic*. It had a harsh, clinical feel to it. "Let me tell you what I have seen that seems to be the kinds of things we expect with Alzheimer's—the more common symptoms."

Both Karen and Lawrence smiled and leaned forward again in their seats.

As I looked at them, the puzzle of Lawrence's behavior did strike me as possibly symptomatic of Alzheimer's disease. This is an illness with many forms, many ways of appearing in the lives of its sufferers. And as I talked to Karen and Lawrence, I tried to capture this quality in my words—tried to draw them a picture in words of the nature of this illness. But it's difficult to do. It is very much like trying to grasp water in the palm of the hand.

Lawrence McGlynn's problems started out as Alzheimer's often does. At first, he had subtle lapses in his memory. He would move from the kitchen of his house to the living room on an errand, and he would forget the reason for his trip just as he arrived in the living room. It happens to everyone, and it was no cause for concern.

But the lapses continued, and became more and more frequent over the months. Lawrence misplaced his car keys, his pen, the newspaper. And slowly, he began to worry more and more about his forgetfulness. Very slowly, a sense of impending doom came over him and began to filter through his thoughts, spreading like some dark-gray blanket over his life.

He hid his worry at first, and made excuses for the forgotten errands and misplaced objects. But as time passed, he found it harder and harder to recall the most basic things. Karen began to notice, and she worried about it as well. The worry and the forgetfulness combined and darkened the blanket, until it became a shroud of depression for Lawrence.

What on earth was the problem? His memory had always been excellent, something he took a great deal of pride in. Now it was crumbling, as much as he tried to conceal it, and life became an effort to hold together—until one day, when Lawrence became lost driving home from the grocery store three blocks from his home where he had shopped, on a weekly basis, for the past ten years.

His wife found him at a neighborhood park, sitting in his car crying while a group of children played on the swing sets in front of him. She drove him home and put him to bed, and the next day, she persuaded him—after a long argument—to go and see their family doctor.

There was confusion at first, and the diagnosis was not clear. Eventually, Lawrence saw a neurologist for his memory problems and he was told, after a lengthy evaluation and testing, that he probably had Alzheimer's disease. Karen had suspected it, but it still came as a shock. Lawrence was having trouble holding on to new information in his thoughts, and this piece was no different from all of the rest.

Karen had noticed that he could remember information from the distant past much better than anything that happened to him recently. It didn't make sense to her. How could he remember his childhood, or details of their life together from twenty years ago, and yet not recall what happened yesterday?

As it progresses, Alzheimer's disease robs people of their ability to function in the present, and so people retreat to the past, to things that are familiar to them. Like Lawrence McGlynn retreating to the parking lot of The Last Call Motel on Aurora Avenue, crouching in the shadows of a pickup truck.

Along with these troubles with memory, and usually well after the onset of the forgetfulness, patients often have difficulties with speaking and understanding people. They can have trouble finding the right word, or sometimes even being able to say what they want to say. The words of their friends and families take on a puzzling form and sometimes become meaningless to them.

It is all a slow, gradual process, and it does not march out in a clear progression through my patients' lives. Rather, it can be a jumble of lost keys and missed appointments and misunderstood messages, a confusion that swells out from the center like air rushing into a balloon, pressing up against all that it comes into contact with.

This is Alzheimer's disease, and what Lawrence McGlynn had experienced fit with this. There could be other things, of course. Intense fears, depression, paranoia, even breaks with reality where people took on strange beliefs and heard strange things. At times, there could be hallucinations.

But not the Cuban baseball team! This did not fit with Alzheimer's disease—these vivid hallucinations Lawrence McGlynn had of these baseball players standing around his bed in his dark bedroom, staring down at him until out he went racing into the night.

Visual hallucinations are usually associated with toxic assaults on the brain, medication side effects, infections, sometimes brain tumors. The vivid, well-formed visions that Lawrence had are not common in Alzheimer's disease. It wasn't out of the question for this to occur—nothing is out of the question with Alzheimer's. But it didn't quite fit.

I leaned forward in the small space and looked at Lawrence and Karen McGlynn. "There has to be something else," I said. "I think we need to make sure something else—a brain tumor maybe, or a small stroke—didn't cause these visions." Karen, who had been listening intently to my words, nodded. "You know, Doctor," she said, "Lawrence grew up in Havana, before Castro came to power. He played baseball there, when he was very young."

Now Lawrence leaned forward and stretched out both hands, palms up. "Look at these hands, Doc. Take a look at 'em," he said. "What do you see? What do you see there?"

I looked down at his rough palms and the deep lines running through them. "I see a catcher's hands, Mr. McGlynn," I said.

115

Lawrence smiled and flipped his hands over, slapping the palms down on the table simultaneously. "Good guess! Good guess!" he shouted. "My first coach down there wanted me to be a catcher, even had me try out for it. But it wasn't for me. It didn't quite fit."

He paused and turned his hands back, palms up, and stared down at them. "I was a first baseman," he said. "A left-handed first baseman."

I nodded. "I'll bet you were a power hitter," I said.

"Batted third in the lineup, sometimes cleanup. If Manny was out, I moved to cleanup."

Lawrence McGlynn's eyes grew larger and rounder, and he looked away from me out toward the door to the room. "Those were great days," he said. "The best of my life."

Karen reached over and patted his arm—once, twice, three times—with her hand. "I wish I had known you back then, dear," she said.

Several seconds passed, as Karen and Lawrence stared at each other in the small office. For an instant, as I watched them, the years dropped away and their faces were transformed into those of the young lovers they had once been. I did not want to speak, did not want to break into their memories of the past.

Finally, Karen turned toward me. "What kind of tests do you want to do?"

Lawrence continued to gaze at his wife. He didn't look as if he had heard her question. I reached out and tapped the back of his hand with an index finger. "Lawrence," I said, "I think we need to get a special kind of X-ray of your head—called an MRI scan—to make sure you don't have a tumor or a stroke in there."

Lawrence looked up at me. "OK," he said.

Now I looked over at Karen McGlynn. "And I also want to get some blood tests, to make sure his electrolytes are normal, that there aren't any metabolic or infectious causes of these visions."

Karen smiled. It was a tight, tense smile. "Do what you need to do," she said.

The magnetic resonance study of Lawrence's head came back normal, except for a few high-intensity signals deep in the brain. The neuroradiologist didn't think they were important, but the technology of the MRI scan is new, and we keep finding things on it that may or may not be significant.

"That's all I see," the radiologist said, "except for the usual atrophy."

I thanked him, and hung up the phone. The *atrophy* he mentioned was a shrinkage, or wasting away, of the brain. As we age, all of our brains lose some of their substance and shrink down a bit. The brain is like any other organ of the body: the lung, the heart, the liver. As we get older, it can slowly begin to shrivel. This wasting away has no direct connection with Alzheimer's disease, or anything else that leads to lost memories and confusion.

The blood work I ordered on Lawrence McGlynn was completely normal. The results didn't help me to find an answer to the cause of his vivid hallucinations. But at least I could tell Mr. McGlynn and his wife that our tests ruled out a few things.

"The good news is you don't have a brain tumor or a blood clot up there," I said. I was sitting in the small interviewing room with Karen and Lawrence McGlynn, going over the results of the tests with them.

"Then what's causing these visions?" Karen asked.

There was an edge to her words, a harsh, quivering sound. Next to her, Lawrence sat up straight in his chair—his back stiff and erect, barely touching the back of his chair. I tried to choose my words carefully.

"I'm not sure what's been causing these visions," I said. "I wish I had an answer for you, but I don't." I paused, to give the words a chance to register. Lawrence smiled at me.

"These visions might be a part of your Alzheimer's disease, Lawrence," I continued. "Or our tests may not be advanced enough to pick up what's causing you to hallucinate."

Karen interrupted me. "But what can we do? He can't just go running out in the middle of the night. He can't do that. Aren't there more tests you can do?"

Karen looked like she was going to cry. Her lower lip was trembling, and she bit down on it to hold back the tears.

Her husband reached out to her, putting his arm around her shoulder. "There, there, little bird," he said. "Don't you worry. It won't happen again."

I took a deep breath, then I tried to answer Karen's question. "I know it's frustrating to hear that we haven't found an answer. But I've started Lawrence on a medication that should stop the hallucinations from coming back."

"What medicine, Doctor?" Karen asked.

"A medicine called Risperdal," I replied.

"What?" she asked.

"Risperdal. It's a new medicine that seems to work well to take away hallucinations."

Karen winced at the sound of the word *hallucinations*. Risperdal was a new kind of medicine, and I was using it a lot with my older patients. It was the same class of drug as Haldol—an antipsychotic with some sedating effects. But it had fewer side effects. People were less likely to become dizzy on it, or to stiffen up like Olive Texas had done. And there was some evidence that it was more effective in stopping hallucinations than the older antipsychotic medications were.

I explained all of this to Lawrence and Karen, and then I went into some detail explaining how it worked in the brain at the neurotransmitter level.

"We think these visions Lawrence is having are related to an increase in levels of a substance that builds up in the spaces between the nerve cells in the brain—something called dopamine." I paused and waited, but there were no questions. "The Risperdal blocks the effects of the dopamine," I said.

Karen leaned forward. "If I understand you right, Doctor, this medicine will block Lawrence's symptoms—these visions he's having—but it won't help us to understand the visions, will it?"

I nodded.

"I mean, that's the problem," she continued. "Maybe there's a reason these baseball players are coming to see him. Why are they appearing?"

She stared at me, and her eyes stretched out toward me like upraised palms. It was a question I dreaded. It was a good question.

"I wish I knew the answer to that," I said. "I wish I did." I turned toward Lawrence McGlynn. "What do you think, sir?" I asked. "What do you think all of this means?"

Lawrence took a long time to answer. Finally, he spoke. "I was a switch-hitter," he said. "Could go either way. Either way."

Lawrence McGlynn's visions did not come back during the time he was in the hospital on our unit. There were other tests we could have performed—a spinal tap, for instance— to see if he had any unusual infections hiding in his brain.

But it really didn't make any sense, and it was unlikely anything would turn up. Mr. McGlynn was discharged after a short five-day stay.

The question Karen McGlynn posed—"What do these visions mean?"—touched at the very core of uncertainty that rests at the heart of Western medicine. We don't know. We don't know so many things. What causes depression? What causes diabetes? What causes rheumatoid arthritis? The questions go on and on, circling inside walls that hide them behind a facade of facts and studies and paperwork, walls that create an illusion of complete knowledge where large gaps exist.

But Lawrence was better, the visions were gone, and I hoped they would stay gone if he kept taking the Risperdal. I scheduled a follow-up visit with Lawrence for a few weeks after discharge, as I wanted to see how he was doing. Then I moved back into the flow of my days, and I didn't think about him further until one day about a week later, when I received a phone call.

I was at the nursing station on our unit when Kristen, the unit secretary, handed me the phone.

"Who is it?" I asked.

"I don't know," she said. "I can't make out what she's saying." Kristen looked concerned.

"Hello," I said. "This is Dr. Mathiasen."

There was a high-pitched sound, like a scream. And then—*"Help me! Help! I think he's dying!"*

I recognized the voice immediately—it was Karen McGlynn. It took a long time before I could understand anything she was trying to tell me. For several seconds, all I could hear was the sound of her breathing rapidly in and out on the other end of the line. And when she was finally able to speak again, her words came out in a rush of jumbled syllables and sentences.

Finally, she was able to tell me that her husband, Lawrence, was lying on the floor of their kitchen. I asked her to check to see if he was breathing. Karen set down the phone. She came back a few seconds later, and now I could hear the relief in her voice as she told me that her husband was breathing, and that she had found a pulse.

Then, slowly, Karen McGlynn told me what had happened. They had just finished lunch and were sitting with their coffee at the table in their kitchen. Lawrence was talking about the upcoming World Series, and he was telling his wife that he thought the Braves' pitching would beat the Indians' hitting. And then he said something that struck her as odd.

Lawrence McGlynn told his wife that he didn't think either team could beat the Havana Blue Devils. It was the team he had played for fifty years earlier in Cuba. The same team he saw crowded around his bed the night before he went into the hospital.

She paused. "And then it happened, Doctor."

"What happened?" I asked.

"He stopped talking, right in the middle of his words. I was watching him over the lunch table," she said. "First he stiffened up, all over his body, like a string pulled tight. Then his eyes rolled up in his head until all I could see was white, and he started to shake."

What she was describing sounded like a seizure. "Could he hear you while it was happening?" I asked.

"I don't know. I don't think so," she said. "He slid down onto the floor, and then his legs and arms started bouncing up and down, and it went on and on, and I thought he was going to die."

She stopped, and I could hear her labored breathing as she cried softly on the other end of the phone line.

Lawrence McGlynn had experienced a grand mal seizure, and it was a frightening thing for his wife to see. I called 911 and sent an ambulance out to bring him in to the hospital. Seizures rob people of consciousness when they happen, and as they regain their awareness they are confused and disoriented. Lawrence was just waking up as he arrived back on our unit, rolling through the double doors at the end of the hall, pushed by a muscular emergency medical technician.

Lawrence was sitting up on the stretcher as well as he could, with his arms and legs tied down to the bed by the leather straps the emergency medical technicians had applied. He looked around, moving his head back and forth until his gaze fell on me. He stared at me, but he didn't seem to recognize me. *"That was foul!"* he screamed out.

By this time, the stretcher had rolled up in front of me, and I stood not more than a few feet away from Lawrence McGlynn.

"You know goddamn well that was a foul ball!" he shouted.

Lawrence was back playing baseball.

"Has he been like this since you picked him up?" I asked one of the men pushing his stretcher.

"Ever since we put him in the ambulance," he said. "He was calling balls and strikes at first. Then it was like a play-by-play of a ball game—I never heard anything like it before."

Lawrence strained to sit up on the stretcher, and the veins in his neck stood out. "I'm tellin' you, that was a foul ball!" he screamed once more.

Then he fell back on the stretcher and closed his eyes. His

body jerked once, twice, in a spasm of movement. Then he was out cold.

What had caused the seizure? Only so many things can happen to the brain to cause its neurons to flare up like dry kindling in the sun. A tumor, an infection, a blood clot, a stroke. Maybe a toxic cause, like a poison or too much alcohol, or sometimes a derangement in the levels of electrolytes in the blood. But I had looked for all of these things on Lawrence's admission to the hospital, and none of them were there. It was unlikely the seizures were caused by Alzheimer's disease alone, as this usually only happened in very advanced stages of the illness.

I repeated the MRI of Lawrence's head, to make sure he hadn't had a stroke or some new damage to the brain. The scan was the same as it had been before. We did a spinal tap, and that was negative as well. There were no signs of infection in his cerebral spinal fluid. His electrolytes and the rest of his blood tests were normal.

I was puzzled. Did Lawrence have something wrong with his brain that our tests couldn't find—that was at a level of resolution that just wouldn't show up on the scans and blood tests? Seizures are not common in the earlier stages of Alzheimer's disease, not something we find very often until late in the illness, at a point when patients have lost most of their language and ability to reason.

Then I noticed Lawrence McGlynn's electrocardiogram from this admission. It was different from his hospitalization of a few weeks earlier. On the tracing now, I saw that his heart was not beating in a regular rhythm. The rhythm had changed, and now the chambers of his heart were each beating on their own, not connecting in a symmetrical fashion. His heart was in a rhythm we call atrial fibrillation.

There are four chambers of the heart: two small ones, called the atria, and two larger ones, called the ventricles. The human heart is driven by electrical impulses, and the impulses connect the chambers so they all beat in a way that moves blood from the atria to the ventricles, and then out through the body and back to the heart. But when something goes wrong, the impulses can be interrupted, disconnected so that the chambers begin to beat independently of one another.

This is what had happened to Lawrence McGlynn's heart. The atria were beating at a much faster rate than the ventricles of his heart. The atria were fluttering, moving in a blur of speed and contracting two or three hundred times each minute like the wings of a hummingbird. Only maybe a third of their electrical impulses were dropping down to the ventricles, to allow the heart to pump blood out to the body. But how did this relate to his seizure?

I wasn't sure. This kind of rhythm—atrial fibrillation— can cause blood clots to form in the heart. The heart beats in such an irregular way that blood can sit in pools in the heart, before it is pushed along, and sometimes clots can form in these pools. Was Lawrence pushing these small clots out into his circulation, and then on up into the brain? Even if he was, it seemed unlikely that the clots were causing the seizures. More likely, they would cause strokes or transient ischemic attacks (TIAs).

I decided to call in a cardiologist to take a look at Lawrence and his EKG. Dr. Jan Curtiss saw him the day after he was admitted to the hospital. Dr. Curtiss is a small woman, about five feet four inches tall. She is an excellent cardiologist with a gruff manner. She took a look at his EKG, and after thinking it over, she said, "Let's send him for an echo, Pat. Let's see if we can find out what put him into A. Fib."

She was suggesting an echocardiogram—an ultrasound image of the heart. It was a simple test, with no real risk to Lawrence. A small transducer would be run over his chest—it would send sound waves down into his heart, and they would bounce back up out of the chest, forming an image of the inside of the heart that we could look at closely. It was a good way to look for any abnormality in the structure of Lawrence's heart, and to see if he was forming blood clots that might be embolizing to his brain.

The echocardiogram showed that Lawrence McGlynn had a large blood clot, called a thrombus, down in the left ventricle of his heart. Though I couldn't be sure, it was possible that pieces of this blood clot were breaking free and spinning out into his circulation and up into his brain, falling into the gray matter like pebbles into water, the waves rippling through his thoughts and bringing forth memories of his youth. It wasn't the most likely explanation, but we had nothing else to explain his symptoms.

Jan Curtiss looked at the results of the echocardiogram. She pointed at the blood clot. "Could that be causing the seizures?" she asked.

I didn't have an answer for her.

I met with Karen and Lawrence McGlynn the next day, to go over the results of my evaluation. Lawrence was more alert and more oriented now. But he didn't recall what had happened the day before.

"Hi, Doc," he greeted me. "I'll bet you didn't expect to see me so soon."

Karen McGlynn didn't say anything. She stared at her husband, with a look of concern on her face. I started right in. "We found something I didn't expect," I said.

I explained to Karen and Lawrence that we had found an irregular rhythm in the heart, and that when we looked further, we found a large blood clot sitting in Lawrence's heart.

"A blood clot?" Karen asked.

I nodded. Karen looked puzzled. "What does that have to do with what's happened to him?"

"I'm not sure," I said. "But I think it might be connected to his visions, and his seizure."

Even as I said it, I knew my explanation was unlikely. Blood clots in the heart rarely led to seizures. But I had nothing else to offer them, and Lawrence was not so advanced in his Alzheimer's disease that I would expect that this alone could be causing his seizures. Karen's voice brought me back to the present. "You think! What do you mean, *you think?* Don't you *know?*"

I spent a long time talking with Karen and Lawrence that afternoon, trying to explain the finding, trying to explain to them why I couldn't be certain.

Many things can cause the heart to beat irregularly, in the rhythm of atrial fibrillation: electrolyte disturbances, thyroid disease, valvular problems in the heart, a blockage in blood flow to the heart itself. It was this last thing that we thought was probably the cause of Lawrence's rhythm disturbance. It was possible that he was flipping in and out of this rhythm, going from a normal heartbeat into the fibrillation and back again. This could explain why it wasn't there on his EKG during his first hospital admission.

"And these clots can cause these visions?" Karen asked.

"I think it's possible," I said.

"But why wouldn't they show up on your brain scan?" she asked.

"On the MRI?"

"Yes," she said.

Sometimes, if the blood clots that traveled up to the brain were small enough, they didn't cause permanent damage. They could splash into the brain and then slowly dissolve. It was possible that this was happening to Lawrence.

"So, what do we do now?" Karen McGlynn asked.

I paused for a moment. "We give Lawrence a blood thinner," I finally replied. "A medication called Coumadin, to break down the blood clot. And we give him an anticonvulsant medication called Dilantin, to stop the seizures."

Lawrence McGlynn stayed in the hospital for another week. During that time, I gave him the Coumadin and the Dilantin. He had no more seizures while he was on our unit, and I discharged him at the end of the week. Lawrence was pleasant through it all, and not especially worried. It was Karen who was anxious.

I had been as honest as I could be with both of them. And along with the honesty came an uncertainty that is a part of medicine, and a part of living with Alzheimer's disease. I didn't think Lawrence McGlynn's visions of the Cuban baseball team, or his seizures, were a part of his Alzheimer's. But only time could tell me this for sure. If I was right, my treatment would likely take away his visions and his seizures.

I saw Lawrence every two weeks for the next several months. He did well at home with his wife. He took the blood thinner and the anticonvulsant medications, and he slept through his nights. Each time I saw him, he greeted me with an exuberant handshake and what became a standing joke between us: "Batter up," he would say.

"Two outs and a full count" would be my reply.

"Runner's going on the pitch! Runner's going!" Lawrence would say.

The visions and the seizures never returned for Lawrence McGlynn. We did a follow-up echocardiogram, and it showed that the blood clot in his heart was gone—dissolved away. I was able to stop the Risperdal, the antipsychotic medicine, and just leave him on the Coumadin and the Dilantin. And Lawrence was able to continue living independently, even as his memory slowly failed.

Why Cuba? Why baseball? These questions troubled me, kept intruding into my thoughts long after Lawrence McGlynn left the hospital. Of all of the stored-up memories of a lifetime coursing through his mind, winding down in among the synapses and nerve fibers like rafts in white water, what was it that had reached into Lawrence and pulled out the visions of the Havana Blue Devils?

We often overlook the "why" in medicine as we focus our attention on the technology at our disposal. But the technology is transient and changeable, while the questions are a constant handed down to us through the centuries.

I decided to pay a visit to Lawrence and Karen, to see if their home could give me any clue to what had happened. The McGlynns lived in North Seattle, in a working-class neighborhood of small houses with immaculately groomed front lawns.

Lawrence and Karen were sitting in the kitchen when I entered. A year had passed, and I didn't know what to expect. Karen beckoned me in and poured coffee. Lawrence sat at the table, smiling.

"Thank you for coming," Karen said. "He's been doing great since he left the hospital. All he talks about is baseball. He talks about it so much, I think he's back there playing it again."

Lawrence looked over at me and slapped the palm of his right hand down on the table. "Batter up," he said, and laughed.

He stared at me, but there was no recognition in his eyes. I looked from Lawrence over to Karen. "I have to ask this," I said.

"Go ahead, ask us anything you want," she said.

"Why baseball?" I asked. "Of all the things in his life, why do you suppose he has held on to the memories of baseball as his other memories slip away?"

Karen's eyes opened wide as she stared at me. "Why, you're the doctor," she said. "Don't you know?"

I shook my head from side to side.

Lawrence stood up from the table and placed his hands one fist over the other, as if he were holding a bat. He spread his legs and swung the imaginary bat back and forth, as if getting ready for a pitch.

"Why," Karen said, "those visions of Cuba and the baseball team are the best thing that ever happened to Lawrence. That was the best time of his life, growing up there and playing ball in that sunny place."

Lawrence called out. "Come on and pitch to me," he said.

Karen went on. "And now he's back there, living through it again. He is truly back there in Havana, and it is a miracle."

"A miracle?" I asked.

Lawrence swung his arms together in a graceful arc out over the kitchen table, and I felt the wind pass over me as his hands passed in front of my face.

"There she goes, Manny! There she goes! *Hasta la vista,* baseball."

Karen smiled as if she had seen this before. "It is a miracle, Doctor," Karen said. "God has reached out and touched him, and He has led Lawrence into a place in his memories where his life has meaning again."

CHAPTER EIGHT

Arrivals

Time floats around the edges of these stories. It is the ocean of time that Mary Pearson's daughter talked about in my office that day. It's difficult to interrupt this flow, to step in and give a definition to Alzheimer's disease. The directions are not clear—too much can blend together, the horizon comes close and then falls away again.

This part of the book examines the lives of four patients who have moved out into their loss of memory and language to a point where Alzheimer's disease seems clear and terrifying. Their stories seem to have more clarity. But do they really?

Images of advanced Alzheimer's disease make us shudder and silently pray that it never happens to us. And sometimes we say it out loud. Sometimes we say, "I'd rather be dead." To outsiders, Alzheimer's is a condition without hope, a malady that strips us of our humanity and leaves us without that thing most essential for us to remain human: our reason.

But this isn't what I hear from the families of my patients. They don't march into my office and say these things. Very rarely do they abandon their loved ones. More often, I'm trying to convince them that they need help, that they need to bring help into the home to bathe and clothe their husbands, wives, mothers, and fathers. Sometimes I have to tell them that they need to find a place for their loved ones to live that can provide the nursing care they need.

People stricken with Alzheimer's disease do not suddenly lose their humanity. I do see pain and suffering, wandering and darkness and shouts in the night. But I see more.

There is the humor that we saw in Lawrence McGlynn and Bridget McNamara. There is a life force struggling up through the depths of Alzheimer's. It struggles and struggles until it breaks the surface and rears its head like a swimmer coming up for air.

Alzheimer's disease reveals many things to me. It can be both touching and frightening, but it is always powerful and I think more than anything else, it has shown me glimpses of the truth hidden down amid its twisting distortions. The illness strips away the social graces—the "Hi, how are you?" questions, when we really don't care—until we come closer and closer to real meaning in our lives.

CHAPTER NINE

The Art Collector

June 17—A good day. Made it to the Carliss show, even talked to a few people. No one suspected.

June 29—Lost on 4th Avenue, missed lunch. What's happening to me? I grew up here. A bad day.

August 14—I smelled baking bread today, like my mother used to bake. Then I don't remember. Nothing!

August 28—I hate Oldenberg. Big baseball bats. Big hanging cows. Big deal.

Samuel Ford was a meticulous, compulsive man, and his traits were reflected in the electronic journal his brother had discovered. Samuel had kept a nearly daily record of his experience from years back as he struggled with his hopes and plans.

Samuel held on to the thread of his good days and bad days through the journal, right up to the last few months when he lost even that, and the words he wrote began to make less and less sense as he fell into waters where his memories ran together like ink on a page.

The journal entries stopped about two weeks before Samuel became lost in Boston. Stopped, as if the journey had come to an abrupt end—skidding to a halt as Samuel found himself unable to type in the words, or even to direct the words in his mind to make sense on the computer screen in front of him. And this is how his brother Arthur found him, staring out at the glowing gray-blue empty screen that sat turned on in front of him in the hotel room on the desolate street in Boston.

Arthur Ford stood in my office as he told me the story of his brother Samuel. He would not sit down, though I offered him a chair several times.

"No thanks," he said. "I've been sitting on the plane, all of the way from Boston." Arthur paced back and forth as he talked. His mouth was curled up slightly at the corners, as if he were in pain.

I had received a call the day before from an internist I knew in Boston, asking me to see Arthur and his brother as soon as I could. The internist had known the family for years, and he asked me to evaluate Samuel when he arrived in Seattle. All I knew was that Samuel had been lost for several days, and his brother Arthur had finally found him wandering the streets of Boston.

Samuel sat behind Arthur in my office, on one of my lavender upholstered chairs. His legs were crossed, and he smoked a long white cigarette that he balanced between his slender fingers. Samuel bore a striking resemblance to Arthur, with the same black eyes and hair. But his expression was different; his mouth was open in a broad and empty smile. He looked as though he did not have a care in the world.

"We're identical twins," Arthur said, gesturing toward Samuel. "Maybe that's what helped me to find him. God knows, I don't know what else did."

Arthur stopped pacing for a moment and reached into his

suit pocket. He pulled out a cigarette, tapped it twice on the back of his hand, and then put it in his mouth and cupped both of his hands around it. In a second, the match flashed and smoke rose through his fingers.

I usually ask people not to smoke in my office. But something stopped me this time. Maybe it was the expression on Arthur's face—the look of pain mixed with fear. He inhaled deeply on the cigarette, then tilted his head back and blew a thin stream of smoke up toward the lights on my ceiling.

"I'll tell you what I know," he said. "At least, what I've been able to piece together about where Samuel spent the last week." He paused and looked at me. "Then you can tell me what you make of it."

Arthur Ford had not been close to his brother over the past twenty years. They had drifted apart, each pursuing his own life and interests. They were both now in their late sixties, and each successful in his own right. Arthur was an investor in stocks and bonds; Samuel was an art collector. They had not seen each other in ten years when Arthur received a call from one of Samuel's clients, telling him that Samuel had missed an appointment and had simply vanished.

Arthur was the only living relative Samuel had. At first, he was annoyed by this intrusion into his life. But he contacted the police in Boston, where Samuel had last been seen. And when they had no idea of how to locate him, he decided to begin his own search.

"I started at the airport," Arthur said. "That's where I got my first clue."

It was provided by a ticket agent who had seen Samuel Ford standing near one of the boarding gates at the airport. The man remembered him clearly, because Samuel had looked confused and lost. He was about to ask him if he could be of help, when he noticed something odd. Samuel was staring right at him, but he didn't seem to see him. Then Samuel began walking toward him. Samuel's eyes rolled up toward the top of his head, and his right arm began to shake and flop out of his control, the muscles moving in spasms from his hand to his forearm to his shoulder. The seizure swept over his brain, the neurons firing wildly, and he couldn't talk—couldn't understand his surroundings. His eyes locked on the ticket agent.

The man told Arthur that he didn't think his brother was really conscious. And as I pieced the incident together later, I thought he was probably right. Samuel Ford was having a seizure, and some primitive part of his brain—lost among the randomly firing neurons—was driving him to protect himself.

He flailed out with his left fist, finally connecting on the third swing, striking the clerk across the temple. Then Samuel spun around and sprinted down the waxed tile floors of the airport, racing out through double glass doors and across the road into a parking garage.

The ticket agent had been taken completely by surprise, and he crumpled to the floor under the weight of the blow to his head. He was not hurt seriously, and he managed to pull himself to his feet and summon security. By the time they arrived, Samuel Ford had disappeared into the parking garage. They searched through it, going over each floor carefully, but they couldn't find a trace of him.

"He was supposed to catch a flight to Zurich," Arthur said. "He bought tickets to Zurich, but he never made the flight."

Arthur Ford's voice wavered as he said these words to me, and I could sense the fear in his voice—a trembling uncertainty. He didn't know what was happening to his twin brother, or how it could be happening. Behind him, Samuel Ford continued to smile the smile he had carried into my office. His countenance was the mirror opposite of his brother Arthur's; at ease, content, safe now that he was sitting in a room with his brother and me.

"You know where I finally found him?" Arthur asked.

He waited, tapping the index finger of his right hand slowly on the top of my hardwood desk—the fingernail beating out a *click, click, click* that rang through the office like a mantra.

I shook my head.

"I found him in a run-down part of town, in a hotel room above a biker bar."

"A biker bar?" I asked.

He paused, and then nodded his head. "The place scared me real bad," he said. "I followed him there through his Visa charges. The hotel didn't take Visa—only cash. But he went to a restaurant next door and used it, and so I tracked him there and then I just started looking around the neighborhood until I found this hotel. The Last Ride, it was called."

Arthur Ford shook his head from side to side. He had been talking rapidly, and there were small beads of perspiration on his forehead above his right eye. He repeated the name of the hotel: "The Last Ride. Can you believe it? Samuel and I never even knew places like this existed when we were growing up."

Arthur told me more about his brother's background. He and Samuel came from a very wealthy family, and neither of them needed to work for a living. Samuel had a degree from Yale in English literature, but along the way, he developed an interest in postmodern art. The interest had evolved into a passion for collecting, for buying and selling and investing in pieces he considered powerful.

Samuel was scheduled to fly to Zurich, to an auction, when he disappeared. It seemed like a sudden event, coming from nowhere to interrupt Samuel's and his brother's lives. But it was not quite that way. Samuel's memory had been slowly failing for months and years, barely noticed by the people around him.

Samuel led a very solitary existence. He had never married, and once his parents passed away, he kept little contact with his brother as he pursued his work of buying and selling art. He had no need to employ a secretary, no need to work closely with anyone else. He liked it that way—traveling from one event to another, making all of the decisions himself. His lifestyle left little opportunity for anyone to notice problems, and even if they were noticed—who would there be to tell?

Samuel's memory had gradually begun to fail. At first it was small things, misplaced appointment books and keys, things Samuel could easily cover. He was not even aware of it at first, until one morning about five years back when he awoke to the sound of a telephone ringing. When he answered, he heard the voice of an angry young artist asking him why he had not appeared for his show.

This jarred Samuel, and he became frightened and worried that something was wrong. So he began recording his thoughts and experiences in the files of his portable computer. This log is what his brother brought in to show me— a computer disk with the words *The Memory Problem* scrawled across the fading paper label. It contained the record of Samuel's failing memory, stretching back five years to that missed appointment with the artist.

It contained the last four entries, from June through the end of August, that appeared on my computer screen when I retrieved the file. Arthur Ford and I stared at the words, and behind Arthur I saw Samuel rise up and move toward my desk. He brushed past his brother and leaned in toward me, reaching for the disk. "I want," he said, "I want mine."

I admitted Samuel Ford to our inpatient unit. There was nowhere that he could live safely, and his thoughts and memories had lost any sense of connection. Now he wandered without direction through the world, seeing and hearing things that seemed new and strange to him, sometimes blacking out with the seizures that came so unexpectedly.

On our unit, Samuel continued to wander—up and down the long hall of gray carpeted floor, from his room to the nursing station and back again. He walked with his head bent forward, staring down at the ground and pulling his long, thin frame along in a steady, relentless way like rain that won't stop.

He wandered through our unit, picking up objects at random, turning them over in his hands and staring at them. Pens and notepads and clipboards. Anything he could find. Sometimes he would stuff the pen or piece of paper into his pocket and stubbornly refuse to give it back.

One day soon after he was admitted, Samuel picked up my tweed sport jacket and put it on. The jacket was draped over the back of a chair behind the nursing station, where I often left it. I was standing by the station talking with Birgitta, one of our nurses, and I didn't pay any attention as Samuel brushed past me, his head bent low, and rounded the corner of the desk. It was only when I heard a shout from behind me that I turned around.

"Hey, hey, hey!"

It was Kristen, our unit secretary, shouting at Samuel Ford. He was standing in front of her, one arm already stretched through my jacket, twisting to fit his other arm into the open sleeve.

"Stop that, Sam!" she said. "Put that back."

But it was too late. He pulled his left arm up and back, and thrust it into the sleeve of the jacket before she could reach him. I heard a dry, tearing sound as the jacket slid up over his arm and onto his shoulder. It was my favorite jacket. "Mr. Ford," I said, "don't do that."

I reached out toward him, but he pulled back—just out of my grasp. Samuel Ford's eyes opened wider, and I saw the dark-black pupils stretch out toward me, surrounded by brown irises. It was the last thing I saw before I felt the blow—his eyes staring out at me like dark canyons.

Something struck the left side of my head, right above my ear, and everything flashed to white in front of me. I found myself rolling forward in a gentle swaying motion, ever so slowly turning over and over, floating out into the air.

What I couldn't see was Samuel, standing above me and watching me fall. But he wasn't really watching me. A fire had started in Samuel Ford's brain, deep down in the temporal lobes, deep down in the folds and convolutions of his mind.

Like a match touching on dry kindling, it had spread as the neurons fired one after another, building on each other until the electrical firestorm moved up to the surface of his brain and out into his hands and eyes and he felt the rush of heat overwhelm him. Samuel stayed on his feet, and he continued to walk toward me. But he had lost the voluntary control of his arms and legs. He was having a seizure.

The fire was raging out of control in Samuel Ford's brain.

It was pushing him to strike out wildly, without purpose, swinging his fists randomly at a world that he could no longer see.

This was the first time a patient had ever hit me. There had been threats before this, of course, and some patients had even grabbed me—my arm, my hand, even the lapel of my coat. But never had a patient punched me like this before.

I remember talking with a colleague several years ago, a Russian psychiatrist who practiced in Moscow. Vladimir told me that under the old Soviet system, psychiatrists were given a higher rate of pay by the state than the other medical specialists. When I asked him why, he looked at me with a puzzled expression. And then, in his best English, he said, "Why, it is more dangerous. We are killed by our patients sometimes."

This concept is not a part of American medicine. But Vladimir's point startled me. I have never been concerned about my safety in the course of my work. I don't ever recall driving to the hospital, thinking about my schedule for the day and wondering if I would encounter any threat. Although I work with patients whose inhibitions are often loosened, with people and families under intense stress who walk at the edge of anger and even rage, I don't spend much time thinking about it.

I am the doctor. As I lay on the floor at Samuel's feet, that was the thought that went through my mind: *I'm the doctor. How dare he do this to me?* In our training as physicians, we are taught to be in control. Over and over in so many ways it is hammered into us that we are the ones who call the shots in all of our encounters with our patients. Finally, this becomes second nature to us and we believe that we can control any situation.

It is a paradox in my specialty that in order for me to hear and understand my patients, I must let go of this control and turn the interview over to them. I must sit back and listen as people explore their anger and fear and motivations, and the better I am at doing this—at relinquishing this control—the higher the risk of my patients touching on something deep and frightening and turning the emotion toward me.

Samuel Ford's fist came up out of some burning piece of his brain—but it didn't matter where it came from. It smashed into the ease and comfort of my days, piercing through my false facade of safety as it crashed into my temple. And it introduced into my life and work an element of fear that has remained there ever since, floating quietly in the background of my encounters.

In many ways, I think this is a healthy thing. I no longer sit down with my patients without, at some level, being aware of the potential danger that lies in the spaces between us. I have developed more respect for the pain—emotional and physical—that my patients struggle against. I am more aware of the unexpected anger and violence that can arise in the course of our talks.

This is a respect for the range of behavior of which we, as all humans, are capable. I do not sit in fear of my patients. I do not believe that psychiatric patients are any more dangerous than other people. But I do think that the nature of my work brings me a little closer to the place we all carry inside of us, the place that wants to lash out at the world around us.

Samuel Ford was having a temporal lobe seizure. These kinds of seizures affect the lobes of the brain that are involved with language, movement, and reason, and when seizures occur in this part of the brain, it often leads to complex behaviors. People can walk, talk, and appear very much alert, and often they become violent for no apparent reason. All of the behavior is without purpose. It is as if the victim is being driven by an unseen hand, possessed in a grip he cannot shake loose.

Were the seizures related to Samuel's memory loss? To his confusion and wandering? I wasn't sure. Alzheimer's disease itself is not associated with seizures, although in its end stages, as the brain crumbles and deteriorates, it can eventually lead to seizures. Is this what was happening with Samuel?

The MRI of his head was negative. There were no tumors, blood clots, strokes, or anything else unusual. It was a clean image of his brain, the gray-and-white matter spread out over the film smoothly and evenly.

I ordered an electroencephalogram next, to look at Samuel's brain-wave patterns. I was looking for an abnormal pattern buried in his brain, down in the temporal lobe region. But it wasn't there. Our neurologist saw only some slowing down of the brain-wave patterns—something that would be expected in dementia. The area around the temporal lobes looked normal.

But it was possible that Samuel Ford was having seizures, and we weren't catching them on the EEG. Pinpointing the origin of seizures can be a difficult thing. They often don't appear when we take an EEG at a given point in time. Normally, I would just treat Samuel with anticonvulsants and see if his episodes, what I thought were seizures, would stop. But this was difficult with Samuel. He was very reluctant to take any medications, and getting him to swallow the anticonvulsant would be a full-time job. Before I committed him to this, I needed to know for sure whether he was having seizures. And so I did something I had never done before with a severely demented patient. I decided to monitor Samuel Ford's brain over a longer period, to see if I could catch the seizures on the tracing at the time they occurred.

This was not a simple thing to do—especially in a patient whose memory and reason were failing. I transferred Samuel to our EEG telemetry unit, and hooked him up to the monitoring equipment. Samuel was fitted with a helmet that was attached to his skull by electrodes, so that the tracing of his EEG could be recorded continuously, twenty-four hours a day. This way, if he had a seizure it would show up on the recording.

Cameras were trained on Samuel Ford wherever he went on the telemetry unit, so that his every movement could be recorded and compared with his brain-wave tracings. If he had another episode of violence, the behavior could be compared with his EEG to see if there was any evidence of a seizure happening at that moment.

It took two days before I finally found what I was looking for. Samuel Ford wandered through the telemetry unit picking up pencils and pieces of paper and everything else he could reach. He took the objects and turned them over and over in his hands, and then he would stuff them into his pockets and not give them back to the staff. But his EEG remained steady and even. There were no episodes of violence.

Then I saw it. It happened just as I was about to stop monitoring Samuel and disconnect him from the recording equipment. He was standing at the telemetry unit nursing station, holding a clipboard out in front of him at arm's length and squinting at it like a doctor making rounds. He pulled the clipboard closer in to his face, and then suddenly his hand opened and the clipboard dropped to the floor at his feet. It bounced back up, and hit him in the shin. But he didn't seem to notice. He continued to stare out at the space in front of him where the board had been.

Samuel Ford's eyes opened wide, wide, wider still as he stared at the air in front of him. Then his right arm, the arm that had been holding the board, dropped down to his side and bounced off of his thigh. On the EEG tracing, the brain waves began to bounce and jump, moving into higher gear like a car engine turning over as it moves into the passing lane. Samuel let out a loud grunt, and he turned back toward the equipment at the nursing station—monitors and electronic recorders and cameras that rested on top of a long counter.

I was sitting just behind the equipment, in one of the chairs at the nursing station. Before I could move, before anyone could move, Samuel's long slim fingers had fastened—one hand on each side—around the uppermost monitor, a silver rectangular piece of metal about the size of a large CD player. On the screen in front of me, his brain waves jumped higher in long jagged spikes that stretched across the monitor.

Samuel pulled back on the equipment in one smooth, quick motion. He ripped the monitor from its moorings, and tiny pieces of metal popped loose from underneath the object and rained down on the desk around me. The screen in front of me went to black as the jagged tracing of Samuel's EEG blinked out as if it had never been there at all.

I looked up from the darkened screen in time to see Samuel Ford raise the piece of metal above his head, holding it high. I thought he was going to throw it over the desk, and I raised my hands in front of my face. But he didn't do that. He stared out at me and at the nurses gathered around the station. None of us could move. We were frozen in the intense light of Samuel's eyes.

145

He raised the object higher and higher, stretching toward the ceiling with it as if holding up a prized possession, like a piece of art that he had bid upon. Then he turned and began to run down the long, narrow hallway of the unit, still holding the monitor above his head. I could hear the *slap, slap, slap* of his bare feet as he ran on the tiled floor, the sound fading as he moved away from us.

We had captured a picture of a seizure in progress. The neurologist could see the abnormal, jagged brain waves down in the region of the left temporal lobe. Samuel's odd behaviors, his compulsive collecting of objects, his random outbursts of violence, were probably all a result of these seizures.

It made sense now. Samuel probably had Alzheimer's disease. But he was also having seizures, and the seizures were triggering his confusion and violence. Were the two related—the Alzheimer's and the seizures? I wasn't sure.

Arthur Ford was immensely relieved to know that we had an answer for what had happened to his brother. I tried to tell him that it wasn't the entire answer, but he interrupted me. "*A seizure,*" he said, turning the word over like a piece of candy on his tongue. "A seizure. You can treat a seizure, can't you?"

I nodded. "Yes," I said, "we can treat a seizure."

I explained to Arthur that we could try to treat his brother's seizures, maybe even clear up some of his confusion, but that this wouldn't restore him to where he had once been. I tried to explain that there were two problems here: the seizures and the Alzheimer's disease. But I couldn't slow Arthur down.

"This is wonderful," he said. "Wonderful. When can you start?"

Samuel Ford was sitting behind his brother Arthur in the

little cubicle where I had brought them to talk. He sat in a large padded wheelchair with a food tray fastened down across his legs. Samuel smiled when I looked over at him. He seemed content. Across his chest he wore a soft mesh restraint that was bound to the wheelchair. Samuel's seizures had become so frequent now, almost constant, that we had to restrain him for his own safety.

I looked back at Arthur. "We can start the medication today," I said.

I treated Samuel Ford with a medication called Tegretol. This is a common anticonvulsant used especially for the kind of temporal lobe seizures that he was having. Tegretol does not work immediately. It takes a week or so to build up the dose in a patient's system, and then another week or two before we begin to see the effects. I explained this to Arthur, and I tried to tell him that there were no guarantees that the anticonvulsant would work. It might, but it might not. Arthur would have none of it.

"What else can we do?" he asked.

As I looked at him, I hoped that we could get his brother to take the medication regularly. He had to, in order for us to see if it would work. And almost miraculously, he did, with the help of our nursing staff. One week after I started the Tegretol, Samuel Ford looked better. He began to eat his meals—something he had not done for several days. He went several hours without one of his seizures. He slept through the night.

In two weeks, the seizures disappeared. There were no more random acts of violence, no more swinging out at people. We were able to remove Samuel's restraints, and he stood up from his wheelchair and looked around the unit as if seeing it for the first time.

Samuel Ford's seizures and violence melted away like an outer garment, like a cocoon, and he emerged calm and steady into the world of our hospital ward. He was still confused. He still had his Alzheimer's disease. But as his rage dropped away, the patients and staff on our unit were drawn to him, much like people had been drawn to him before the onset of his Alzheimer's disease.

I couldn't explain it, but I was drawn to Samuel Ford as well. He couldn't communicate with me, at least not in words. But there was something soft and gentle and knowing about him. Something that had not been there before, when he was having the seizures. Now it emerged, and I could feel it in his presence.

Samuel still walked through our unit, picking up objects and examining them, turning the pens and pencils over and over in his hands like things he had never seen before. But now, when staff asked him to return the objects, he gave them back easily.

A few of the other patients on our unit began to follow Samuel on his walks up and down the hallway of our unit. They were the most demented of our patients, and they moved along with Samuel as if pulled by an invisible string. The patients seemed calm in his presence. But still, Samuel did not talk.

On the day that Samuel Ford was to be discharged, I could not find him. His brother Arthur had managed to locate a fine adult family home in North Seattle, owned by a young couple who seemed committed to working with people with Alzheimer's disease. And Samuel seemed to like the place when he went there for a visit.

But I couldn't find Samuel on the unit. He wasn't in his

room. He wasn't in the dining room. He wasn't in any of the other patients' rooms, either. I began to worry. Had he run off?

The questions were bouncing up and down through my mind, and my thoughts were racing as I took one more look in a group room at one end of our unit. It was empty. And then I looked outside the unit. I disarmed the alarm on the door at the end of the hallway with my key and walked out into the rest of the hospital. And just as I passed through the doorway, I heard laughter.

I looked down the hall and saw a crowd of people—four or five—standing bunched together. In the center of this group I saw Samuel Ford's head, with his clear features rising above the others. And as I looked closer, I realized that they were all patients from our ward.

I had no idea how they could have slipped through the door without triggering the alarm. But there they were, surrounding Samuel Ford. I walked closer, to get a look at whatever it was they were staring at on the wall.

It was a print, an Impressionistic painting of water lilies. As I approached, Samuel pointed at the painting with the long slim index finger of his right hand. "Boring!" he said loudly.

It was only the second time I had heard him speak. He waved his right hand dismissively at the painting, turned on his heel, and brushed past me as he walked away.

The crowd of patients stood silent for a moment. And then, almost as one, they raised their hands and waved them in disgust at the painting—in exactly the way Samuel Ford had done.

When Samuel's brother arrived to pick him up, I told him what had happened. Arthur Ford laughed out loud. "He

149

always hated anything that looked like Monet," he said. "Just hated it."

Arthur took a deep breath, and tried to control his laughter. "He would say, 'Those damn lilies.' Right in the Met, with a crowd of people around him. He wanted his art to be alive."

Now the laughter had stopped, and Arthur Ford's eyes grew larger. "He wanted his art to shout and bray at the world. For a moment there, it must have come back to him," he said. "He must have known what he was looking at."

Arthur was crying now, and the tears streamed in tiny rivulets down over his cheeks as he pulled in the air in big breaths and remembered his brother as he had once been.

CHAPTER TEN

Only the Ice
of Death

Many of my patients reach out for beauty, much like Samuel Ford had. And as their Alzheimer's disease progresses, this impulse continues to exist and give meaning to their lives.

Mario Russolini was admitted to our unit one winter day in December, at a time when the rain in Seattle is at its heaviest—pouring down day after day until the low-lying farms and fields around the city flood as the rivers overrun their banks. It's also a time when the days shorten, squeezing down until it is light for only a few hours each day. Into this Mario arrived, accompanied by his daughter.

Mario lived with his daughter and her husband. His memory had been failing, and he had been having more and more trouble with his day-to-day life. But this wasn't what brought him to the hospital.

One night, he awoke to a noise. He listened carefully, and he thought he heard footsteps down in the kitchen. Mario believed someone had broken into the house. He slid out of his bed and crouched down beside it, hiding behind the edge of the mattress. He listened carefully, heard the sound of breathing, then saw a shadow in the doorway to his bedroom.

Mario didn't move. He waited, waited, and then when the shadow moved into his room, Mario finally leaped. He felt his right hand connect with the shadowy figure as his knuckles pressed into something soft. There was a scream, and then bright light flashed into the room, blinding him.

Mario held up his hand to shield the light from his eyes, and slowly, the scene came into focus for him. There at his feet lay his beautiful daughter on the white carpet of his bedroom, with a thin trickle of blood streaming from her nose. In the doorway, her husband stood with his mouth open, his hand still resting on the light switch.

Mario Russolini was a big, robust man with a barrel chest that sat perched atop his narrow hips and skinny legs. He had grown up in Italy, south of Naples in the hills along the Amalfi coast. His father had been a fisherman, and he had been able to make a living for his family. But it had been Mario's father's dream to come to America, and when he couldn't realize the dream for himself, he passed it on to his son.

Mario came to America in his early twenties, not speaking a word of English. He learned the language and created a life for himself here—opening a garage and going on to open several more. But he never lost his connection with Italy. When his wife died ten years ago, Mario retired, selling his business and taking some time to visit his childhood home in the hills along the Amalfi coast.

Mario's daughter told me all of this on the day that we admitted her father to the hospital. Her lip was still swollen, and her right eye blackened from the force of the blow that her father had delivered. Beneath the bruises, she was a beautiful, dark-haired woman with brown eyes and an easy smile.

"He didn't mean to do this to me," she said. "He was frightened."

Her eyes opened wide, and she looked at me with a pleading look. She kept looking at me, until I finally nodded.

"I don't know what's wrong with him," she said, shaking her head from side to side. "I just don't know what's wrong with him."

She stared down at the floor at her feet, and then, softly, she began to cry. I held out a tissue and pressed it into her hand. It took her what seemed a very long time to compose herself.

Finally, she looked up at me and tried to smile. Her lips curved upward in a small, strained arc that stopped—frozen—halfway up her face. "He's lived with us for so long, Doctor, that I didn't even notice it. It was my husband who noticed."

"What did he see?" I asked.

"He told me, 'Your father is forgetting things, Gina.' And I would get mad at him, and tell him he was imagining it."

"What kind of things?"

"Oh, I don't know," Gina said. "Like his keys—he started to forget his keys all the time. He had never done that before in his life." She drew the tissue across her eyes, blotting out some of the tears. "We think it started maybe two years ago. The keys. He would come back for the keys. Then he got lost driving every once in a while. He wouldn't be able to find where he was going, and he would come back so mad and try to hide it from us."

"How did you find out?" I asked.

"His friends would call, and ask us where he was." Gina shook her head again, and her long dark hair swung in an arc above her shoulders. "But it was so slow. So slow at first, if my husband hadn't said anything, I never would have noticed. And it was only in the past six months that my husband began to talk about it."

"The past six months?" I asked.

Gina's cheeks turned red. "I'm sorry," she said. "I'm sorry. I know I should have taken him in to see a doctor sooner." She took a deep breath, and her shoulders rose up around her neck as her voice rose in the room. "But I couldn't," she said. "I just couldn't." She looked around, as if frightened by the sound of her own voice. Then the words spilled out in a torrent like rain. "He's my father and I love him and he lives with us, and there just couldn't be anything wrong with him."

The tears came again. She held her arms straight out toward me. "He's my father!" she cried out. "He's my father, and you have to help him! He can't find his way on walks through our neighborhood anymore. He gets lost. If we buy new furniture, it throws him off and he bumps into it. And now look what he's done."

She pulled her right arm back and pointed at her swollen lip. "Look at this. This isn't him. He would never do this to me." She stared directly into my eyes. "Please help him," she said. "Please help him. I don't know what to do. I can't take him home, the way he is now."

Gina's words ran through my head as I left the small consulting room and walked slowly back to the ward: *I don't know what to do.* I had heard the same thing from many families of patients suffering from Alzheimer's disease: *What can we do? What should we do?* I still wasn't sure I had a good answer.

I did think Mario Russolini had Alzheimer's disease. It all fit. The gradual loss of memory. The forgetting, the confusion, the striking out at a world that made less and less sense.

But Mario's evaluation had been done in a piecemeal way, and as I looked for him on the unit, I knew I needed to pull the threads together, to make sure I wasn't missing anything.

A family physician had diagnosed depression, and there probably was an element of this, especially at first when Mario began to misplace his keys and to lose his way. As the realization that something was going wrong began to sink in, Mario did become depressed. But then it went beyond this, as Mario's confusion rose up in front of everyone around him.

What was wrong? Gina took her father to a neurologist, who thought the blanks in his memory, his becoming lost in the streets, might be due to seizures that Mario was having. The neurologist thought Mario might have had a small stroke, or even a brain tumor, that created a focus in the brain from which the seizures could start.

He ordered an MRI of Mario's brain, and it was completely normal. No stroke. No tumor. Then he did an EEG: again, normal. And finally, a spinal tap looking for signs of infection. But again, nothing.

All of these thoughts were passing through my head, along with Gina's words, when I rounded a corner and heard the laughter. I looked up and saw Mario Russolini leaning up against the nursing station, his elbows resting on the top of the counter. He was gazing up at Birgitta, our Swedish nurse, and laughter was rising from his chest.

Birgitta is a striking woman, young and tall with long blond hair and an easy grace. Mario leaned forward on his elbows, his eyes spread open wide like moons, and he stared up at her with a silly smile on his face. The laughter stopped for an instant, and then I heard the words rise deep from Mario's chest: "*Ah! Soltanto il nostro fuoco spegnerà di morte il gel.*" (Ah! Only the ice of death can extinguish our fire.)

155

And then again: *"Ah! Soltanto il nostro fuoco spegnerá di morte il gel."*

Mario was singing from the Italian opera *Lucia di Lammermoor,* although I didn't know it at the time. Birgitta laughed and pushed on Mario's forehead with the palm of her hand.

"You are a wild man," she said in her Swedish accent. "Wild."

Mario Russolini pushed himself back from the counter with both hands, until he was standing straight up. Then he bent forward and with a flourish swept his right hand out in front of him, bowing to the young woman standing in front of him. For an instant, I saw Mario the young man appear, standing in one of the coffee bars in his hometown of Ravello. The smile spread across my face, and I could not help but laugh as I watched him.

I was still smiling as I walked up to Mario. He held out his hand to me, and I took it reflexively. Mario pumped my hand up and down two, three, four times with a strong squeeze of the fingers.

"Mario," I said, "how are you doing?"

His smile spread wider across his face, and he jabbed with his index finger at the air. *"Lucia di Lammermoor,"* he cried out. He stared up at my face, searching for something, then let go of my right hand. "Lucia," he said. "Lucia."

I nodded my head slowly up and down, but Mario knew I was trying to fool him. He shook his head back and forth with anger. "Gaetano Donizetti."

I finally had to admit it. "I'm sorry," I said. "I don't know the opera."

Mario took a deep breath, and his chest rose up against his hospital pajamas. *"Congiunga il Nume in ciel"* (Let God unite us in Heaven), he sang out in his deep bass voice.

It was a lovely sound, deep and rich. Now all of the nurses behind the counter had stopped what they were doing and were watching Mario. His chest puffed out again, and the words came forth.

"Se divisi fummo in terra, ne congiunga il Nume in ciel . . ." (If we were divided on earth, let God unite us in Heaven . . .)

Mario stopped singing, but the words stretched out over the nursing station and on into the dining room. Down the hall, many of my patients came out of their rooms to see what was happening, and as I watched they gravitated toward the sound that still wavered in the air like fresh-cut flowers.

In front of me, Mario Russolini knelt down at the counter where he had been standing. I thought he was bowing again to Birgitta, but he bent until his knees touched the floor, then he swiveled around and plopped down in a sitting position.

This is where he stayed, his back pressed up against the wall of the nursing station, unwilling to move, seemingly unable to hear us as we implored him to rise. And on his face was a half smile and a look in his eyes as if he saw something far away that none of the rest of us could see.

Soon after this, I met with Mario's daughter and her husband in the small conference room on our ward. Mario joined us, and all three leaned forward expectantly, waiting to hear my news.

"Thank you for coming in today," I said.

As I looked at each of their faces, I found myself wishing I had something more certain to tell them. Only Mario smiled as he leaned forward, and he was the one who spoke first. "Lucia," he said. "Lucia."

I smiled back at him. "I read it, Mario," I said. "A beautiful opera."

Mario nodded his great head up and down several times. Then his mouth opened and he sang out, *"A te vengo— o bell' alma . . ."* (I am coming to you—O beautiful spirit . . .)

Mario looked at me, and I knew I had to answer him. *"Pensa al ciel,"* I sang back. (Reflect upon Heaven.) *"Pensa al ciel."*

It was the line that stuck in my thoughts, after reading the opera: "Reflect upon Heaven." My wife found the libretto for *Lucia di Lammermoor* buried at the bottom of an old cardboard box in a corner of our basement. As I read the words from the libretto I thought of Mario and how he had been captivated his entire life by the two doomed lovers in the story. And somehow, the words rose up off the yellowing pages and took life, and for the first time in my life I wanted to see an opera.

Mario leaped to his feet, and his two hands—big and thick and heavy—swept out in front of him in wide arcs, crashing together once, twice, three times.

"Bravo!" he cried out. "Bravo! Bravo!"

Mario's daughter, Gina, stood up and walked over to her father. She reached out and took his hands in hers.

"This was—is his favorite opera, Doctor," she said, turning toward me. "He sang it to me and to my mother over and over as a child, until I know it by heart."

Gina's eyes glistened under the fluorescent lights in the room, and she looked away. "I have not heard him sing it in a very long time," she said softly.

It was quiet in the room for a while, and I waited. Finally, Gina's husband broke the silence. "Could you tell us what you've found, Doctor?" he asked.

This is the question I dread with Alzheimer's disease. I want to be able to tell my patients and their families things with certainty. I want to give them a clear idea of what to expect from their illnesses. But with Alzheimer's disease, all of this goes out the window. It is an illness marked by its uncertainty and unpredictability, and when I try to apply the words of Western science to this disease, the words just don't sound right.

"Well," I started, "I've reviewed all the tests that have been done—the MRI and the CT, the spinal tap, and all the blood work."

Gina looked back up at me, her dark eyes wide now. She nodded her head eagerly, and Mario next to her mimicked the movement with his own head. I went on. "Everything looked good," I said. "There's no evidence for any treatable causes of Mario's memory loss."

Gina interrupted me. "Is that good?" she asked. "I mean, wouldn't it be better to find something you *could* treat?"

I smiled. Gina was pointing out one of the great ironies of Alzheimer's—it can only be diagnosed by ruling out other illnesses, and even then, we can't be certain.

"You're right," I agreed. "I do want to find something we can treat. But your father hasn't had a stroke, or a brain tumor, or an infection in the brain that's causing his confusion. So in that way, it's good news."

Gina helped Mario to sit down, and then she sat down next to him. "So what is it?" she asked. "What's causing this?"

Next to Gina, Mario leaned back on the small couch and put his arm around her shoulders. He pulled her toward him, and squeezed her tightly.

"We did one more test," I said. "A SPECT scan."

"A what?" Gina asked.

"A SPECT scan—a test to assess the function of your father's brain. The letters stand for *single photon emission computerized tomography.*"

"It's a test that, well, it's not specific for Alzheimer's disease, but it has some findings that are . . ." I paused. The words *Alzheimer's disease* were hard for me to say, and now that they were out in the room, they hung in the air like a strong odor. Gina and her husband looked away, and only Mario kept staring at me. On his face a look of concern appeared as he frowned and his eyebrows pushed in toward the top of his nose.

". . . that are suggestive," I continued. "That's what we found, a pattern suggestive of Alzheimer's," I finished the sentence awkwardly.

Now the silence grew stronger in the room. Still there were no questions. Gina began to sob quietly, and Mario tightened his grip around her shoulders. I waited. And waited. Finally, Gina's husband spoke, as he had before. "So, Doctor, do you think Mario has Alzheimer's disease?" he asked.

I took a deep breath, and then another. I was glad the question was finally out, where we could all hear it, see it, almost reach out and touch it. "As I was telling you before, this is a diagnosis—"

Before I could finish my sentence, Gina broke down in loud, shaking sobs. They were guttural sounds, rising from somewhere deep in her chest, and the sounds frightened me. I stopped and looked at her.

Gina slowly regained her composure. The sobbing subsided, until she stared out at me with her hands raised in front of her. "What do you think it is?" she finally asked. "I know you don't *know* for sure. But what do you *think* it is?"

Gina's husband reached over and put his hand on her arm, trying to steady her. Now they both looked at me—waiting. I took one more deep breath.

"I think Mario probably has Alzheimer's disease," I said. "Everything points toward it. The history, the tests, the—"

Then I noticed that Mario was not looking at me any-more. He was looking across the room at a Monet print hanging on the wall. And I was talking about him as if he weren't sitting in the room. "Mario," I said. "Mario?"

His head swung around and he looked at me. On his face I still saw the knitted brows above his eyes. "Mario," I said, "I think you have a disease that makes it hard for you to remember things. That's why you're here, in the hospital."

Mario's brows knitted down tighter above his eyes, until his eyes almost closed in a squint. I wasn't sure that he had been able to understand me. I was about to repeat myself when he spoke.

"Can I stay with Gina?" he asked.

There was a pleading tone to Mario's question, and his eyes opened wider as he looked up at me, his face opening up like the palm of a hand reaching out. I looked at Mario for what seemed like a long time before I answered.

"Mario," I said, "I think you need to move into a place where you're safe, a place where your family doesn't have to worry about you."

"What kind of a place?"

It was Gina asking the question. She had shaken loose from Mario, and was on her feet in front of the couch. "What do you mean—'a safe place'?"

Gina's husband stood up beside her, and for the first time, I noticed his features. He was a tall, muscular man with a long torso and bright, piercing green eyes. His nose was long and slender, coming to a point on his face like a hawk.

"Honey, you know he's right," he said. "It's just not work-ing at home anymore. We can't keep taking care of Mario."

Mario stood and walked slowly toward his daughter and son-in-law. He stopped directly in front of them, and I wasn't sure what he was going to do. He just looked back and forth, from the face of his daughter to his son-in-law and back again. For an instant, I thought he was going to strike out at them.

Gina moved first. She reached out with her right hand, the palm open, and touched the side of Mario's face. She held her hand there as she spoke. "I'm so sorry, Dad," she said. "I don't know what to do."

The tears came, welling up from her chest into her eyes and falling into the room in a shaking sob that spread from Gina to her husband and then to Mario. Then the three closed together, hugging each other tightly, Gina and her husband pulling Mario in until he was obscured from my view and all I could hear was the sound rising from a circle of tears.

The crying went on for a long time, seconds, minutes, several minutes, interrupted only by the sound of air rising in and out of their lungs as the three people breathed. And then, from the center of the group, I heard Mario's voice softly: "It's OK, Gina," he said. "It's OK."

With the help of our social worker, Gina found Mario an adult family home in which to live. It is a wonderful place, a big rambling 1920s house in the Queen Anne neighborhood of Seattle with four other aging residents who needed some help in life. And best of all, it is run by a tiny Italian woman—Maria—who, along with her husband, helps these five to get by, and does it with a flair and a belief that the infirmities of old age are no excuse for bad behavior.

Mario grew to love this place. Maria would give him a little wine, she would play her operas for him, and she and her husband would sit down with him and watch soccer games on their cable television hooked up to the huge silver satellite dish that stared one-eyed up at the sky from their roof.

I heard no more from Mario until I received a card one day in the mail. It was an invitation to a birthday party—Mario's birthday party.

The Pink Door is an institution in Seattle, an Italian café hidden down in the winding streets of the Pike Place Market, with a terrace looking out over the rooftops onto Elliot Bay. This is where Mario Russolini's birthday party was held.

I arrived late, and I found the entrance to the restaurant in the narrow alley behind the place, right across from the Pike Place medical clinic where I had worked years before. The door was painted pink, and it was fading in places where the paint had chipped off.

I walked down the two flights of stairs into the restaurant. It was dark inside, and I squinted to see as my eyes adjusted to the light in the room. I squeezed past the tables in my path and climbed up the steps that led to the terrace where the party was being held.

Up ahead, several tables crowded together under hanging flowers and plants. The bright light from candles and lamps encircling the squared-off veranda shone into my eyes. Mario's family had rented the entire terrace, and in the center of the tables I could see a huge birthday cake with candles—dozens of candles—ablaze on top of it. There must have been forty or fifty people crowded around the tables, all of them looking toward the bay that spread out down below.

I tried to see what everyone was looking at, but again, it took a minute for my eyes to adjust to the sudden change from darkness to bright light. I put my hand up to shade my eyes, and slowly, the scene came into focus.

Up at the front of the terrace in front of an iron railing, Mario stood next to a tall blond-haired woman. It was Birgitta, the nurse from our inpatient unit. Behind them I could see Elliot Bay stretch out from the port of Seattle, reaching out into the deep dark waters of Puget Sound. Light hit the waters of the bay, shining down from the city and bouncing off the smooth surface like shiny silver streaks of paint.

Mario bent down in front of Birgitta, sinking onto his knees and gazing up at her. I could see her smile at him, and then his voice boomed out, and from where I stood at the back of the terrace, I could hear the words he sang as clearly as if he were standing right next to me.

"Ah! Soltanto il nostro fuoco spegnerá di morte il gel." (Ah! Only the ice of death can extinguish our fire.)

The words hung in the air, echoing out over the terrace. And for the first time, I noticed the moon big and full and round floating out above the bay.

Mario stood up and I could see his eyes open wider and wider, shining as they looked out over the crowd. For an instant he was home once more, a young man looking out from the streets of his village down into the waters along the Amalfi coast. And then the crowd of birthday guests were on their feet, applauding and shouting the words "Bravo! Bravo!" out into the night.

CHAPTER ELEVEN

Sleeping Beauty

Alzheimer's disease suspends patients in time, cuts them off from their surroundings and leaves them adrift in the minutes and hours that make up their days. But it is not the only disease that does this.

Mona Lokal sat propped up in her bed at a forty-five-degree angle at the Sunrise of Life nursing home, and stared at me where I stood at the foot of her bed. Actually, she stared out into the space in front of her, her gaze unwavering. I just happened to be standing in a position where her eyes met mine. If I moved a few steps to the left, or to the right, her eyes would not follow me. They remained locked onto an imaginary point in the air.

I had been asked to consult on Mona. She was an old woman in her eighties, and everything had been tried. The long line of specialists—the neurologists, neuropsychologists, internists, pulmonologists, gastroenterologists, and even the dermatologists—had trooped past the foot of her bed and stood exactly where I stood. The tests had all been done, the patient examined. And all of the specialists had nodded their heads and agreed: There was nothing else they could offer.

This was dementia—probably Alzheimer's disease. But

Mona's daughter, Shirley, wanted one more opinion. She pushed and pushed and pushed until Mona's family physician, Dr. Alex Landry, gave in and called me.

I spoke to him one morning, and he told me about this patient he followed in the nursing home. She wouldn't eat. She wouldn't speak. She was slowly dying, and he didn't know why.

"Will you take a look at her, Pat?" he asked. "The family is going crazy, and I'm going to have to give her a feeding tube if she doesn't eat something real soon."

"Sure," I said. "I'd be glad to see her."

Mona Lokal looked very frightened as I watched her face from the foot of the bed. Her eyes were open wide, with thick black eyebrows pushed up above them, wrinkling her forehead into deep folds of skin.

Mona Lokal did not speak. She did not communicate with people in any visible way. She had been eating less and less, until now, she was not eating at all. Visitors came by rarely, and Mona Lokal was essentially cut off from the rest of the world.

This is one of the great fears of people as they grow old— to be left alone by those they have loved. It does not happen very often. But sometimes it does, as it had with Mona. Her life had become so filled with pain that the pain spread out to those around her, pushing them away like a great muscular arm until they could no longer come close to her.

Mona had been this way for two years. And now that she had stopped eating, her condition—whatever it was—had become life threatening. I looked at her and tried to decide how to begin.

"Good morning, Mrs. Lokal," I said. "How are you doing today?"

She continued to stare straight ahead, out into the space in front of her. She did not blink, and I looked into her green eyes trying to find a sign that she recognized my words. But there was only the green surrounding the small black pupils. I reached down and gently rocked her right foot from side to side with my hand.

"Mona," I said. "Can you hear me?" There was no response.

"You might want to try leaning right down by her ear and talking real loud, Doctor. That used to work sometimes."

I whirled around, startled by the voice. In the doorway to the room a heavyset black woman stood with her arms folded across her chest. "I'm Arlissa," she said. "I been working with Mona for a few years now."

I nodded. "Thanks. I'll give it a try."

I walked around to the head of the bed. Mona Lokal's gaze did not waver. She continued to stare straight ahead as I bent down until I was close to her left ear. "Mona," I said in a loud voice. "Can you hear me?"

Again, no response. No indication my words had registered. I put my hand on her shoulder and rocked it back and forth. Still nothing. I looked up at Arlissa. "How long has she been like this?" I asked.

Arlissa shrugged. "Seems like forever," she said. "I know when I started working here a year ago, she was eating a little bit. But even then, she didn't talk much to any of us. And since that time, it's got worse. Do you think she has Alzheimer's?"

"I'm not sure," I replied.

"That's what everyone thinks. But it don't look like no Alzheimer's to me."

"Why not?" I asked.

The woman looked surprised. "Well, if you want my opinion, most of the old folks we got here with Alzheimer's,

167

they don't look like Mona. Their memory starts to go, but they keep talking to us and they keep eating. It's only at the end, when their mind goes, that they stop those things."

Arlissa smiled. "But I ain't no doctor," she said.

"No, no," I said. "Please go on."

Arlissa took a deep breath. "Well," she said, "this all happened too fast to Mona. Alzheimer's is slow and easy. But the charge nurse here, she tell me this started happening to Mona in just a couple of months."

"A couple of months?" I asked.

Arlissa nodded her head.

I looked back toward Mona Lokal. She lay still in the bed, staring out at me as she had before. What was the problem? Was this Alzheimer's disease? Was it something else?

I walked back over by her bed to look at her more closely. As I watched, I thought again about the patients Oliver Sacks wrote about in his book *Awakenings,* the frozen ones with post-encephalitic Parkinson's disease who sprang to life with the wonder drug levodopa. If there were only a magic pill for Mona—a way to bring her back from this floating, suspended death she had embraced.

I reached down and touched her hand. There was something about Mona, something that made me want to reach out and touch her. I didn't understand it. She was all but dead, almost gone from this world. There was nothing in her yellowing skin, or the pained expression on her face, that would make me want to reach out to her. And yet, it was there—coming up from somewhere deep inside of her. She was cut off from the rest of the world, yet I could feel her reaching out toward me, trying to meet my touch.

Could she have advanced Alzheimer's disease? I didn't think so. There was something in Mona struggling toward the surface, like a swimmer in heavy waves. Although her features were rigid and still, I could feel the tension rising and falling inside of her. This was something different from Alzheimer's. I could feel the give-and-take of a fight going on behind the grimace etched into Mona's face. And I thought, for the first time, that the fight might be with depression.

Out at the nursing station, I looked through the chart rack until I found Mona's chart. It was thick, stuffed full of sheafs of papers and laboratory results and nursing home forms, all together making up the bureaucratic paper trail that the state demands of these facilities. Mona's chart was the largest at the Sunrise of Life nursing home. I took it over to the counter, set it down with a heavy thud, and flipped it open. It took me a few minutes to find what I was looking for: the neurology evaluation.

Mona had been seen about a month earlier, and by the description in the neurologist's notes, she had looked the same then as she did now. He described her wide-open eyes and the expression of fear on her face. I read quickly through his notes, skipping ahead to his impression: "Dementia— probable Alzheimer's type."

This was his primary diagnosis. This was what he felt was the cause of Mona's behavior. The neurologist talked about the possibility that her difficulties were the result of other illnesses—perhaps a stroke, a brain tumor, a chronic infection of the brain. Not once did he mention the possibility that Mona might be depressed. But this is what I kept thinking of as I looked through the lab results and printouts, the exams and the opinions.

The diagnosis of Alzheimer's disease had been made. And once it is made, it sticks tightly to the patient. It cannot be removed. But the diagnosis didn't quite fit. Mona's decline had been too rapid, she had shut out the rest of the world much too quickly for this to be Alzheimer's. I agreed with Arlissa, the aide. This did not fit with a dementia.

Depression can be a mask that appears as Alzheimer's disease. There is even a term for it: We call it *pseudo-dementia.* Something that seems to be a gradual loss of memory and intellect, but is really a loss of interest and the will to live. A person's spirit sags and he or she slowly gives up on life. But how can we tell?

Sigmund Freud talked of depression as anger turned inward on the self. Freud was a neurologist before he became a psychoanalyst. He understood that there are many physical causes that lead to depression. But Freud also understood that depression can lead to physical problems. This was one of his great discoveries—that emotions could be expressed as physical illness.

There was no blood test I could do to confirm my suspicions. Depression, even more than Alzheimer's disease, is a diagnosis based on history. And the person who could tell me the history—Mona—was not able to talk. Arlissa had given me some background. But I needed more. I flipped through the chart until I found the name of Mona's daughter, Shirley Lokal. She lived in the Seattle area, and next to her name was a telephone number. I picked up the phone and punched out the numbers.

Shirley Lokal picked up on the third ring. She was glad that I had called, and she told me how frustrated she had grown over the past several months as she tried to talk with first one, and then another, of her mother's doctors.

"I couldn't get an answer out of any of them," she said. Her voice hit a high-pitched level, like a piece of machinery grinding on metal. "None of them would call me. And when I would get ahold of one of them, I couldn't make sense out of what they were saying."

I tried to interrupt her. "I'm sorry to hear—"

But she would have none of it. Her words increased in speed, like a ball rolling downhill. "Oh, I know it's not your fault. You called me. You're gonna talk to me. But these other doctors—it was all long, long words and no answers."

She paused, and I saw my opening. "Ms. Lokal," I started, "I'd like to ask you a few questions about your mother. I think she might be depressed."

"What?"

"If you think back, can you remember how your mother's problems started?"

I heard a long, slow sigh of relief almost like a moan coming through the receiver. "Yes. Yes, I do remember how this started. I've been trying to tell all of those doctors, but not one of them would listen to me."

Shirley Lokal went on to describe to me what had happened to her mother. She told me that at first, her mother became nervous and restless. She couldn't sit still. Not at all like what I was seeing now. Then she had more and more trouble sleeping, and her appetite—which had never been good—fell away to almost nothing. Shirley Lokal described an anxious woman who became more and more anxious, pacing through her tiny apartment aimlessly.

"Then she got paranoid. I would go to see her and she would be hiding behind the door, and sometimes she wouldn't let me in."

"I see."

"And she started telling me her insides were rotting away, and she just knew it was true. She would call me to tell me

171

that. It got so bad, we took her to her family doctor—Dr. Russo."

"What did he say?"

"He gave her some Valium, and he told her to stop worrying so much."

"Was she having any trouble with her memory?" I asked. "Would she forget where she left things, maybe leave the stove on, anything like that?"

I was searching for the short-term memory loss that is so common in Alzheimer's disease. There was a long pause on the other end of the phone line, and then the voice returned hesitantly. "No, no, I don't think so," Shirley said.

"Are you sure?"

There was another long pause. "Yes, I'm sure. I'm sure," Shirley Lokal replied finally.

"Did she seem confused at all?" I asked. "I mean, did she ever have a hard time adjusting to new places? Did she ever get lost?"

"No, I don't think so, Doctor," Shirley said. "You have to understand, I wasn't around her all the time. But her troubles weren't really like that. It was more like she gave up on life, but real slowly, until one day I just found her in bed and she wouldn't get up."

"Is that why she had to come to the nursing home?" I asked.

There was a cracking sound on the other end of the line, and then I could hear Shirley Lokal crying into the phone. She was crying so hard, I could barely make out her words as she told me that this *was* the reason her mother had entered the nursing home.

When Shirley finally regained her composure, she told me more. She said that Mona's mother—her grandmother—

had suffered from bouts of depression so severe, she had been hospitalized in state hospitals for months at a time. The episodes were called "nervous breakdowns" when Mona was growing up. And one of Mona's brothers had committed suicide, after years of depression.

Depression, much like Alzheimer's disease, can be hereditary. It had run in Mona Lokal's family, and it put her at a higher risk for it. But was she depressed? Was this what had pushed her into her bed, unable to speak, unable to eat, staring wordlessly out at the world as if she had already passed out of this existence, leaving only the shell of her body behind?

I walked back to Mona's room from the nursing station. As I entered the doorway, I heard a creaking sound. I looked over at Mona, hoping that she was moving. But she wasn't. Mona had not moved from her position in the bed. Next to her bed, a window swung slowly back and forth, caught in the rhythm of a soft wind.

Mona Lokal was slowly dying, as sure as if she had a malignant cancer spreading through her body. It was worse, in a way, because there was no clear illness to attack, no tumor to cut away, no mass to hit with radiation and chemotherapy. There was just Mona slipping away—starving because she was unable to eat.

Mona Lokal was beyond the help of all of the specialists who had seen her. Depression is a real thing. A deadly thing. It was obvious psychotherapy couldn't help her. Even our best antidepressant medications were of no use—Mona was not eating or drinking, and she would not take anything by mouth. As I stared down at her, I could think of only one thing that could hold out any hope of helping her: electroconvulsive therapy.

I watched the movie *One Flew Over the Cuckoo's Nest* as a teenager in the early seventies, and I saw Jack Nicholson—strong, rebellious Jack—tortured by an evil society bent on breaking his will. The evil took the form of shock treatments, given over and over to stop him from freeing all of the patients from the control of the nurses and doctors. The movie left me with an ugly image of electroconvulsive therapy that has stayed in my mind through all of these years. And the image contrasts with my belief that, for some of my patients, only shock treatments can bring them back from the black void of their despair.

Patients have been abused by electroconvulsive therapy in the past. At times, it has been given indiscriminately to people, sometimes even to punish them. But it has also saved lives, as surely as emergency surgery has saved lives. I have no doubt of this. I have seen it work over and over with patients so depressed that nothing else could help them.

Electroconvulsive therapy was discovered by a chance observation more than fifty years ago when a psychiatrist noticed that a patient with schizophrenia—not depression—seemed to improve after he had a seizure. The patient had epilepsy, and each time he had a seizure, his thoughts became more focused and his mood improved. It was a great observation.

Two Italian psychiatrists—Ugo Cerletti and Lucio Bini—went on to develop the technique for the treatments. Electroconvulsive therapy (ECT) is a simple procedure. The idea is to cause a patient to have a generalized grand mal seizure. At first, the treatments were done at the bedside, without anesthesia, and this is where much of the stigma of ECT comes from—the images of patients strapped in their beds, writhing as the electricity is passed into their brains and the seizures occur.

Over the years, the treatments have been refined. Now patients are given a short-acting anesthetic agent so they have no memory of the treatments, and the violent contortions of limbs are controlled by a muscle-paralyzing drug. Electroconvulsive therapy takes place in an operating room, and the risk to the patient is very low.

ECT is now used mainly to treat depression and occasionally to treat manic and psychotic episodes that do not respond to medications. The treatment still carries with it the dread that *One Flew Over the Cuckoo's Nest* tapped into. People are afraid of it. They are afraid of losing control. They are afraid of brain damage, although there is no evidence of any permanent memory loss. They are afraid, I think, of an assault on their brains—and of the potential for losing some piece or pieces of their personality in the process.

We do not understand how ECT works. There are many theories, but after more than fifty years, we just don't know. We do, however, know that 70 to 80 percent of severely depressed patients will get better with a course of anywhere from eight to twelve treatments given over a three- to four-week period.

I only recommend ECT to severely depressed patients who have not, or cannot, benefit from anything else. It is something I would want for myself if I were suffering from a bad depression. This is what I told Mona Lokal and her daughter, when I talked to them about the procedure. And I hoped that Mona's daughter could hear what I was saying.

Shirley Lokal was uncertain about electroconvulsive therapy for her mother. "Are you sure? What if it makes her worse?" she asked.

We talked about it for a long time on the phone. Shirley

was her mother's power of attorney, and since Mona was unable to make any decisions, the responsibility fell to her daughter.

"Why don't you think it over," I said. "And if you have any questions, just give me a call."

I gave her my direct pager number and hung up the phone. Shirley called me back later that afternoon.

"Doctor," she said, "if you think this might help my mother, let's go ahead with it. She looks terrible. She looks like she's going to die."

We wheeled Mona Lokal into the small, bright room early one summer morning. She did not move her head, or even her eyes, as we pushed her on the stretcher through the small doorway. Her face was still set frozen in her terrible scream of fright—like some horrible sleeping beauty awaiting a kiss.

The stretcher slid into place, and one of the nurses—Mary—locked the wheels in place with a loud click that echoed in the space. Pieces of machinery loomed up around Mona. On one side, the ECT equipment sat on a cart stacked like stereo equipment. On the other, the anesthesiologist's array of gauges and monitors sat encased in black like an air-traffic controller's panel. The nurse, the anesthesiologist Dr. Ken Tyson, and I were in the room with Mona.

Ken Tyson was busy getting ready for the procedure, moving among the wires and gauges of his equipment. I had worked with him on many patients in the past. He had a young face, very young, almost boyish in appearance, without a trace of beard or mustache. Everyone called him Kenny.

"Is this her first treatment?" Ken asked.

"Yeah," I said. "First one."

I looked down at Mona Lokal. She continued to stare out, now straight up at the ceiling.

"Mona?" I said. "Can you hear me?"

No response.

"We're going to try to help you with these treatments, Mona." I said the words slowly, in a loud voice. "Mona, we're going to help you to go to sleep. And then we'll give you the treatment, and you'll wake up in a few minutes. Do you have any questions for me?"

I felt silly asking the question, but I felt that I had to. Mona stared silently up into my eyes.

"Ready to go, Pat?" Ken Tyson asked.

I looked over at him, startled by the sound of his voice. The fluorescent light in the room fell evenly over everything, like a bar at closing time when the lights suddenly come on.

"All set," I said.

The anesthesiologist took a syringe and injected the anesthetic agent into an intravenous line running into Mona Lokal's arm. Then he dropped a plastic mask down over her face, covering her mouth and nose, and began giving her some oxygen. Still, Mona did not move.

Ken looked up at me, his smooth skin gleaming in the light. "She always like this?" he asked.

"Pardon me?" I said.

"Does she always look like this? I've never seen anyone look like this before."

"I know," I said. "I know."

As I looked down at Mona Lokal, I felt the doubt pass through me like a cold winter morning. Was this depression? I wasn't sure. Much as I would have liked to be, I just wasn't sure if that's what I was dealing with. Was it worth the risk? What if she had Alzheimer's disease—these treatments might only make her worse, only cause her to become more and more confused.

Mona Lokal was asleep, though it was hard to tell looking down at her. Kenny pulled out another syringe and gave her the muscle-paralyzing medication succinylcholine. In a moment her breathing stopped, and Ken turned toward me. "Go ahead," he said.

Speed was important now. Mona could not breathe on her own, and I needed to give her the treatment—and cause the seizure—as quickly as I could, so the anesthesiologist could go back to supporting her breathing. I had the two electrodes in my hands, "paddles" that carried the electricity from the machine into Mona's brain. I bent down over Mona Lokal.

Different theories exist about ECT. Some people place the paddles on either side of the head, in the bilateral position, and some start in the unilateral setting—with the paddles on only one side of the head. There is some evidence that the bilateral placement leads to a quicker response, a lifting of the depression faster. On the other hand, the unilateral setting leads to less confusion and disorientation as the treatments progress.

With Mona, I chose the bilateral setting. I wanted to get the quickest response that I could, given the level of her depression. I held out the black-handled paddles and looked for the areas, above and behind the corners of Mona's eyes, where I wanted to put the stainless-steel discs that pushed out from the ends of the paddles. I found the spots, and pushed the shiny discs into them.

"Everybody clear," I said.

I looked around the stretcher. Kenny, the anesthesiologist, had backed away and was watching from a point in front of his black instrument panel. The nurse, Mary, was on the other side of me, near the ECT machinery. It was silent in the room, and I could hear the faint *tick, tick* of the clock on the wall above my head.

I looked down at the black paddles. They were in place. I slid my right thumb up over the handle of the paddle in my hand, until it came to rest on the red button that rose up like a flower out of the blackness of the right paddle. I waited for a second, and the silence deepened. Then I pushed the red button deep into the paddle.

Nothing happened for a second. Then two seconds. I held the button down, and I looked into Mona Lokal's face—still frozen in its unearthly pain. And then Mona's features leaped into motion.

Mona's forehead crinkled up into hard ridges of flesh, as her eyes—which had been open up until this time—pulled shut into tight lines below her eyebrows. The corners of her mouth shot out into her cheeks, and her jaws snapped down hard on the rubber mouthguard that rode between her teeth. The skin on Mona's neck tightened into long cords, like rope, and her head arched back until her head pushed into the pillow.

Mona Lokal remained like this for several seconds, as the silence deepened in the room. This was the tonic phase of the seizure, the part where the electrical storm in the brain shoots out to all of the muscles in the body, freezing them in place. The muscle-paralyzing agent, succinylcholine, cannot block this effect completely; it only dampens it.

I looked down at Mona's left leg, where I had placed a tourniquet to stop the flow of blood into her foot. I did this to block the succinylcholine from reaching down into her left foot, so we could watch the effects of the seizure in the foot. The idea was to paralyze all of her limbs except the foot, to limit the risk of injuries, but still give us a chance to witness the seizure and make sure it happened.

Mona Lokal's left foot began to shake, first in very fine, almost imperceptible tremors, then shaking more and more until it was bouncing up and down. I looked up at her head. It, too, was starting to rock back and forth, and the tension from the muscles in her face came together in a tight vibration, like the string of a bow whirring in the air after the arrow leaves it.

This was called the clonic phase of the seizure. I wanted it to last a half minute or more—the length of time that was needed to get a good response to these treatments. Ten seconds passed, and we all—Kenny Tyson, Mary, and I—stared up at the clock. Mary started to count out loud: "Fifteen seconds," she said. "Twenty."

Now we all joined in, like a chorus. "Twenty-five, thirty, thirty-five."

The seizures started to slow. The jerking movements in Mona's foot began to slow, and the spasms of the muscles in her legs became visible. Mona's foot moved back and forth slower and slower, in larger arcs of motion. I looked up at her face. The tension had gone out of it, like air from a taut balloon, and now Mona's neck relaxed and her head bent back on the pillow. The seizure was over. Mona's body sagged out across the stretcher. Her eyes remained closed, and the skin of her face sagged as well, collapsing in a mass of unformed flesh.

On the morning of the second treatment, Mona Lokal was wheeled into the small room on her stretcher. She stared up at the ceiling, not acknowledging any of us.

"She isn't any better," Mary said. There was a low sound, the sound of disappointment, in her voice.

But on the fourth treatment, Kenny Tyson noticed a difference in her expression. "She looks a little better today, Pat," he said.

I looked down at Mona and nodded. Her eyes were not quite so wide, and now her mouth was closed so that I couldn't see her teeth.

"Mona, how are you doing today?" I asked.

There was no answer as Mona stared out at me, but I thought—maybe I was fooling myself—that I saw the curve of her mouth twitch in the direction of a smile. It fell back as suddenly as it had come, back into the lines of her face.

On the seventh treatment, there was no doubt. Several nurses were gathered around Mona in the small ECT room when I entered, and there was a hum of conversation. At first, I couldn't see Mona's face—obscured by the backs of the nurses.

Mary pulled on my hand. "Dr. Mathiasen, look," she cried out as she pulled me toward the head of the bed.

Mona's face popped into view, between the scrub suits of the nursing staff. I didn't recognize her right away. I looked down at her face, and I thought I was in the wrong room. I thought I was looking at a different patient.

"Doesn't she look wonderful?" Mary asked. "I can't believe she's smiling."

And then it hit me. Mona Lokal was smiling up at me. Gone were the painful stare, the stiff and rigid features, the look of horror. In their place was a small, but very real, smile. "Good morning, Doctor," Mona said.

On the ninth and final treatment, Mona Lokal's features split into a wide grin and her face leaped into the room, bright as light passing through a skylight on a clear summer day. She reached out and took my hand as I bent down above

181

her stretcher: "God bless you!" she said. "God is so good to me. He's so good to my family."

Mona's smile stretched wider and wider.

"Mona, how are you feeling today?" I asked her again.

The answer came back almost instantly. "Why, I feel wonderful. Everyone's been so good to me here. But how long have I been here?"

"Mona, you've been depressed. Very depressed, and you're just coming out of it," I said.

The smile dropped away from Mona's face, and she frowned. "That's what everyone keeps telling me. But I don't remember. I don't remember."

And then the frown vanished, and once again Mona Lokal's teeth flashed white behind the curve of her smile.

Mona had little memory of her depression and the way it had held her to her bed in its tight fist of hopelessness. But she realized that she felt better, that in the place of the vast emptiness inside of her, there was now a vibrating energy that she had not felt in a very long time.

"Doctor, I don't know how to thank you," she said to me.

Mona Lokal and her daughter were sitting in my office a few weeks after Mona had finished the course of electroconvulsive treatments. Shirley Lokal smiled, and looked over at Mona. "I can't believe it!" she said. "I can't believe it. I keep thinking I'll wake up." She took a deep breath. "I keep waiting for somebody to pinch me and then I'll wake up and none of this will be true. Tell me it's true."

Mona Lokal started to laugh, at first with little giggles that grew and grew, until she was rocking back and forth in her chair. Her daughter looked over at her.

"What's the matter, Mom?" she asked.

Mona Lokal was barely able to get the words out between the laughter. "I feel so good, honey," she said. "I feel so good."

Shirley Lokal's smile grew wider, and then she, too, was laughing.

The elderly suffer from the stigma of old age. At times, they are patronized, winked at with knowing smiles, dismissed by those of us who should know better.

This is what happened to Mona Lokal. It was no great insight of mine that helped her. It was the persistence of her daughter, who felt that things just didn't add up. It was the observations of Arlissa, the aide who had seen enough of Alzheimer's disease to know that what Mona had just didn't fit. Perhaps it was Mona herself, who held on tightly to life as the parade of specialists trooped by her bed.

Depression is a deadly illness, every bit as lethal as cancer or heart disease. It is something that can be treated, something from which people can recover. But only if it is recognized. Only if we think of it, as we work with our patients in the course of our days.

CHAPTER TWELVE

My Babies

Laura Sunday sat surrounded by her two sons in my office, strapped into her wheelchair and breathing heavily. She picked at her hospital gown with her right hand, while all of the time her head swiveled back and forth—scanning the faces of her two sons—Sidney and Jay.

"Where are my babies?" she asked.

She nearly whispered the words, and I had to lean in close to hear what she said. Then she repeated the phrase, much, much louder: "Where are my babies?"

The sound startled me, and I jumped back from the wheelchair. Laura Sunday looked up at me, and down in her mouth, I could see her thick red tongue moving up and down, pressing up against her teeth like a small animal trapped in a cage.

Laura Sunday was a patient I saw in consultation two years ago. Her older son, Sidney, had called me and asked if he could bring her in. He had been referred by his mother's neurologist, who felt that she might be depressed. When he described his mother on the phone to me, I was left with the image of a woman who was aging and feeling a bit low about the way her life was going. I was not prepared for what rolled into my office that day.

Laura's memory had been slowly failing for several years—her thoughts and feelings gently crumbling like a piece of bread between the fingers. She had had an extensive workup by her neurologist, and by the time she arrived in my office, all of the MRIs and blood tests and EEGs had been done. Nothing reversible had been found, nothing treatable.

Laura's neurologist had given her Cognex (a.k.a. tacrine) for a time, and her sons told me that it had helped her memory at first. This is a medication that is aimed especially at the memory loss of Alzheimer's disease, and it works—at least in theory—by enhancing the presence of the neurotransmitter acetylcholine in the brain.

Acetylcholine, or the depletion of it in the brains of patients with Alzheimer's disease, is associated with the loss of memory. And Cognex does seem to slow this memory loss—at least early on in the illness. Early on. That is the key.

This is what happened to Laura Sunday. She had improved for a time, maybe five or six months, and it was a wonderful time for Laura and her family, a time of hope and looking toward the future. But the time had passed, like a cruel hoax, and then Laura began her slide back down into the dark waters of her thoughts.

Was Laura Sunday depressed? That was the question her sons carried into my office. And as I looked at Sidney and Jay, I realized it was not a simple question. Could this woman be depressed—the way Mona Lokal had been depressed? Maybe that was it. Maybe that was the cause of her confusion and pain.

I didn't think so. Laura's history was classic for Alzheimer's disease. And Laura was not showing the usual signs of depression—the poor sleep and appetite, the lowered energy, the reduced activities. I thought depression was unlikely—but I didn't know for sure. So I admitted Laura Sunday to our inpatient unit for an evaluation.

Sidney and Jay were devoted to their mother, each in his own way. This was one of the things they had in common. The other thing that they had in common was their hatred for each other. These two facts colored their every movement around their mother, their every action with her and each other.

The roots of their hatred ran deep, and they talked about it openly with me. They told me more than I wanted to know. Both of them should have been successful in life. Neither of them was.

Jay was a young man, a thirty-five-year-old internist who really didn't like the practice of medicine; his dream had been to be a poet, but he had been afraid to show any of his writing to anyone. And Sidney was a forty-five-year-old executive stuck on one of the bottom rungs of the corporate ladder at the huge insurance company where he worked. His dream had been to be a cowboy on a ranch in Montana—but marriage, kids, and a house got in the way of all of that.

Maybe fear was another common thing these two carried with them. They had each been afraid, for different reasons, to try to do what they'd dreamed of doing. And now they both felt it was too late, and each blamed the other for his failure.

Jay told me that Sidney had never respected him, that he had always questioned his manhood and his ability to do things. Jay remembered the long nights when his much older brother had dragged him out into the garage beneath the car hood, then had him bend down above the engine and hold

the light in his cold hands as Sidney worked on the car—
every so often growling, "I can't see. Give me some more
light." The minutes ticked by endlessly, like time standing
still, as Jay stood in the garage and tried to pretend that he was
interested in what his brother was trying to teach him.

And as he grew older, his resentment grew as well. It grew
when his brother made fun of the books he read, books by
Camus and Dostoyevsky. It grew when his brother interrupted him in the middle of a book of poetry he was reading,
grabbing it from his hands and tossing it on the couch.
"Come on," Sidney said, "I think we need to replace the
alternator on the Dodge."

Jay hated it. He hated the message that the only real,
worthwhile things were tangible objects of metal that stood
idling in the garage. He hated it so much that it still puzzled
him why, when he entered medical school, he chose the specialty that more than any other area of medicine required its
practitioners to carry in their heads an encyclopedic knowledge of disease and apply it to the human body the way a
very good mechanic would apply his knowledge to an ailing
car engine. He had become a mechanic of human illness.
And he was no good at it.

Sidney's anger was closer to the surface, more obvious
than Jay's. He felt that he had done all of the right things in
his life, and he listed them for me. He had worked hard, finished high school, and then gotten a job in construction. He
worked seven days a week, ten hours a day, in order to save
enough money to put together a down payment on a house
and move his young family out of their basement apartment
and into the safety of the suburbs.

But his brother did not respect him, and he knew it. Jay
could not understand Sidney's motivation—his world

looked foreign to him, and he wanted nothing to do with it.
And he let Sidney know it. From Sidney's vantage point, Jay
had had everything growing up. He had been favored by
their parents, both the mother and father. Jay didn't have to
work, like Sidney had. And when Jay finished high school,
they sent him off to college.

Now Sidney and Jay had little to do with each other,
although they lived in the same city. In fact, they had not
talked to each other in several years, and they told me that
they had stopped—as if by mutual agreement—sending
each other Christmas and birthday greetings about three
years ago.

At first, they felt a gap, a space where each felt the absence
of the other. But this faded with time, growing dimmer,
dimmer, like a porch light burning out. When they arrived
in my office with their mother that day, it was the first time
they had seen each other in three years. Their father had
long since died, and they had carefully timed their visits to
their mother's house to avoid each other.

"You bastard! Why didn't you tell me there was something
wrong?"

Sidney Sunday was standing up on his feet, shouting at
his brother in the small conference room where the three of
us sat around a circular table. I had admitted their mother to
our psychiatry unit, where she had been for the past week.
Sidney and Jay had come to see me to get an update on her
condition. But the meeting had taken a different turn.

Sidney's face was dark red, almost purple in color, and the
veins were standing out on his neck and forehead like knotted pieces of string. He slammed his fist down on the table,
and the sound rang through the room from wall to wall.

"For Christ's sake, you're the doctor," he said to his brother.

I held up my right hand, but before I could speak, Jay had leaped to his feet with his arms raised. They stood on opposite sides of the table from each other, and for an instant, I thought that Jay was going to lunge over the table at his brother. But he didn't. He straightened up to his full height and stared at his brother, and when he did speak, it was slowly, in a low voice. "I'm sorry you couldn't figure it out for yourself," he said. "But then, you never could figure things out very well, could you?"

Jay and Sidney stood staring at each other across the table, and there was a pause in their argument, a small space of time that I leaped into.

"Stop," I said. "Stop it right now. You're not helping your mother with all of this." I pointed at the door with my right hand. "She's out there on our unit, trying to understand what's happening to her. And all the two of you can do is fight with each other."

But neither of them stopped. They had only paused for air, and now Sidney spoke again—this time softer.

"I should have sued you last year, after you suggested putting her in a nursing home. A nursing home, for God's sake. She used to tell me, over and over, that she'd rather be dead than end up in one of those places."

Jay rolled his eyes toward the ceiling of the conference room. It was a dramatic movement, his whole head arching back along with his eyes until he was looking straight up at the tiles on the ceiling, ignoring his brother. And then he turned his back on Sidney. And I heard him say quietly, almost too quiet to hear: "It's too bad you weren't around when it still meant something. When she still knew who you were. You must think she put you in her will."

Sidney's face turned darker and darker, and his lips twisted up in a contorted grimace, like a strange smile. He raised his right arm and began to climb up onto the round smooth table that stood between him and his brother. And it was then that we heard the sound, coming from a long way off: *"Babies . . ."*

We all stopped to listen.

"Where are . . ." There was a long pause. Five seconds, ten seconds, fifteen. Then it came again. ". . . my babies?"

It was Laura Sunday, outside the conference room on the unit, repeating the only words she seemed able to say. Now the sound became clear and distinct. "Where are my babies? Where are my babies?"

Jay spun around from the wall he was facing, and he and Sidney charged past me—nearly knocking me down—as they rushed out the door and into the hallway. I followed them through the swinging door, trying to keep my balance in their wake. And there in front of us, walking slowly behind a metal walker in front of a young man who was guiding her along, was Laura Sunday. Sidney reached her first.

"We're here, Mom! We're here. It's Sidney."

Jay joined him at his side, and reached out to take Laura's arm. "We're here," Sidney said again. "Are you in pain, Mom? What's the matter?"

And in that instant, both sons were transformed from the cold angry warriors that had squared off in the tiny conference room. Sidney's face had lost its dark color. Jay's sneer had dropped away. And they stood on either side of their mother, wanting to help in any way that they could.

Laura Sunday looked from one side to the other, her head swiveling back and forth as first she looked at Sidney, and then at Jay. Her head moved slowly on top of her gray shoulders, and her mouth twisted up at the corners in a smile. "My babies," she cried out. "My babies."

Jay and Sidney stared down at her from each side, watching her every move. They were smiling, too. Everything was quiet in the hallway, except for the sound of Laura's voice. It was much softer now—"My babies. My babies."

Alzheimer's disease can bring families together. And it can push them apart. It brings out the good and bad in our relationships, and it holds these qualities up for us to see. The view is not always pleasant, but it is intense—like a hot ember smoldering deep in our relationships with one another, flashing up at unexpected times to ignite our deepest emotions.

This is what Laura Sunday did to her sons, Sidney and Jay. As her memories slowly receded and she drifted farther and farther out into the waters of her disease, she tried to hold her sons—her babies—close to her. And the closeness touched them, and they were pulled back into the conflicts of a time many years ago; time swallowed them up and they fought like two children together in a sandbox.

Alzheimer's disease can pull us like a black hole into contact with one another. In this contact, there can be anger and frustration, and even hatred, as Sidney and Jay experienced. But there can also be kindness and laughter, and sometimes the realization of love.

I am not immune from all of this. As I watched Jay and Sidney hover near their mother in the hallway of our hospital unit, peering down at her, I thought back to my childhood and my trips with my father to visit his sister—Annana—in the nursing home where she sat in her wheelchair. I thought about the long, bumpy rides in the sun-warmed Dodge, my father's hands tight on the steering wheel.

And then I was there—staring down into the face of the kind old woman strapped into her chair. But it wasn't the old woman I remembered so clearly. No. It was my father who came flooding back to me now.

I remembered again how the visits to the nursing home to see his sister on Sundays had been something I had looked forward to. He would tell me stories of his work on the drive to the nursing home—stories of the railroad, the grease and sweat, and of the men who worked there with him.

He would tell me of how he would go to visit his sister Anna, before she became sick. She lived near the yardhouse where he worked, and he would drop in on her for lunch. In my father's eyes as he talked I could see the tears rise almost to the surface. His sister never turned anyone away, he said, not even the hobos who tromped up to her door in the thirties—during the Depression—looking for food or work.

Our visits to see Anna pulled emotions up out of my father that revealed him to me. And always, each and every time at the end of our visits, back in the car and riding home he would look over at me and pass his hand through my hair, back and forth, back and forth. He would look away, out the window of the car at the passing street, and then the tears would appear on the tanned skin of his face.

Then one day, our visits fell away and stopped. It had become too painful for my father to see his sister as her Alzheimer's disease passed over her, too painful for him to look into her clear, blank eyes. I missed the visits. At first, I thought it was because I missed seeing my aunt. It was only years later that I realized that that wasn't it. It was because I missed the closeness to my father that her existence had brought into my life.

All of this passed through my mind as I watched Jay and

Sidney attend to their mother in the hallway of the hospital. Alzheimer's disease is a powerful illness, and it affects everyone who comes in contact with it—sometimes in unpredictable ways.

Laura Sunday had let go of her four-wheeled aluminum walker and was standing straight up now. Sidney supported her right arm, and Jay held on to her left. It was quiet for a moment, and then Laura smiled.

She pulled her arms free from her sons, first the right and then the left. It was a gentle movement, almost a shrugging of the shoulders. Then she reached out and clasped their hands in hers, Sidney in her right hand and Jay in her left. Her sons looked puzzled, but neither tried to pull away from Laura Sunday.

She held tightly to the right hand of each son. Then, slowly but firmly, she pulled her sons' hands in an arc out in front of her. Laura Sunday kept pulling and her sons' hands moved toward each other out in front of her, closer and closer until the hands touched together, still held firmly in Laura Sunday's grip. Then she let go of the hands and looked from Sidney to Jay.

Jay and Sidney looked up and their eyes met. Gone was the anger and hatred now, and in its place they smiled at each other. Then they began to laugh as their hands came together and they clasped each other in a firm grip. The laughter mixed together in the air with Laura Sunday's words: "My babies. My babies."

CHAPTER THIRTEEN

Hope and Forgetting

Imagine entering a strange, dark room. This is what Alzheimer's disease is like. This is what I dream of when I close my eyes in the silence late at night.

The doorway looms up, and then I am through it and feeling my way along the walls. I reach out with my hands in front of me, waving them to the left and right, feeling for a light switch I can't find. Something strikes my right shin sharp and hard, and the pain shoots up my leg like a long needle and I cry out.

I can't see anything. I squint, but all that appears is more blackness, as if a dark cloak has been thrown over my head. I keep waving my arms and walking slowly, with tiny mincing steps, into the darkness. There is no light switch. No candle. Nothing to illuminate the room.

Fear flashes in my chest like a spark, and in my mind the darkness takes life in a myriad of forms. Mario and Mona and Laura Sunday appear—all standing in the room staring out at me as I grope my way toward them. Samuel Ford and Bridget and Norman Brown, Olive and Mary Pearson, and all of the rest packed into the tight space of the room, watching me as I stumble forward.

My dream recurs, over and over, and I wake up frightened in the darkness—trembling into the silence of the night.

Alzheimer's disease touches on our deepest fears. The fear of losing control. The fear of losing our minds. The fear of becoming something not completely human as those around us watch helplessly. These fears are perhaps stronger than the fear of death, for Alzheimer's disease is viewed by many of us as a walking death, a disease that strips us of all of the things that make us human.

The fear touches me, as it touches my patients and their families. Many of my colleagues look at me in a puzzled way—wondering why I have chosen to spend a large part of my professional life in the middle of all of this fear and confusion. Why?

The answer is not simple, as Alzheimer's disease itself is not simple. As a physician, I have developed the ability to hold most of my patients at arm's length—to keep them at an emotional distance, which allows me to work with them without getting caught up in the vortex of their pain. All doctors do this. We all have our shields, our ways of protecting ourselves.

It doesn't always work. Pain and anger and fear work their way through the shield at times. But there is also hope and laughter and joy, yes joy, that seeps through.

In my own family, there was a silence that surrounded Alzheimer's disease. It really wasn't understood then as Alzheimer's disease. And it affected my father's brothers and sisters, and maybe my father himself.

There was silence because the disease was not understood. And along with the silence came a sense of shame, a suggestion that the victims of this disease had done something wrong, and that maybe, although no one ever said it, the illness was contagious and its victims needed to be isolated.

My father managed to overcome his fear. He would not back down from it. He took me on his visits to see his sister, to talk with her and take her gifts, to treat her with respect as this horrid thief of memory slowly robbed her of her thoughts.

It was only later, in my teens, that I discovered that two of my father's older brothers suffered from this illness as well. They lived a long ways away, in California, and I had never met them. All of his siblings had been affected by what I now believe was Alzheimer's disease.

And it was only much later that I began to see the signs of it in my father himself. Or at least, thought that I saw the signs of it. During my first year of medical school, I began to notice his lapses in memory. At first, it was small things. He would be going to the refrigerator, and then forget what he wanted to eat. My mother was more concerned than anyone else. In fact, she would call me and tell me about it, her voice trembling with uncertainty. "It's starting," she would say. "It's just like his sister." And I would try to calm her down. "Don't worry," I would say in my new professional voice. "Don't worry, Mom, we all do that."

But she did worry. And I worried as well. I called home more often, to see how he was doing. I visited frequently. And I noticed lapses in my father's memory which seemed unusual. He would forget what he was saying in the middle of a sentence. He would forget the names of people he had worked with all of his life. Something did seem wrong.

And then he was gone, taking everything but the puzzle along with him. One bright summer morning, the phone rang into the quiet of my apartment and I picked it up to hear my mother's voice on the other end of the line.

"There's been an accident," she said.

Her voice was strangely calm, her words clear and still traveling down through the receiver into my ear. "There was a storm," she said, as if telling me what she had had for dinner the night before. "Roy was fishing and the wind came up, and they couldn't get out in time." And now her voice caught, but for only an instant and then she went on. "Your brother's OK, but your father—he couldn't get out."

There had been a freak storm, rising up out of the North Dakota plains and sweeping over the reservoir without warning. My father and brother were out fishing in their fourteen-foot aluminum boat, and they had only a few minutes to see the sky darken above them before the winds fell on them and their boat was tossed back and forth like a toy in the whitecaps.

They were separated in the water, and when the sun rose the next morning and the waters finally calmed, he was gone. They found my father's body a few hours after my brother was rescued—floating peacefully only a few hundred yards from where their boat had overturned.

So the puzzle remained. Did he have the Alzheimer's disease that had affected his brothers and sisters? Would it have descended on him like the wind in that reservoir if he had lived long enough to encounter it? I didn't know. I really didn't.

With my mother, it was different. Many years after my father's death, she would look at me and with that strangely calm voice that she spoke in soon after the accident she would say to me, "I miss him, Pat. But thank God he didn't have to suffer like his sister did." She would shake her head slowly from side to side. "That was horrible, what Anna went through. You remember her, don't you?" My mother shook her head again. "Poor woman. It makes me wonder if there is a God."

Louise Billings sunk down into my office chair, down until she was nearly swallowed up by the shades of purple in the upholstery. She had come in with her granddaughter, June, a pretty young woman who sat in the chair next to her and smiled at me. Louise spoke first. "Where am I? Where am I, June? Is this your office?"

June reached over and patted her grandmother on the arm. "We're in the doctor's office," she said. "This is the doctor, Grandma."

Louise Billings's head swung slowly around toward me, until our eyes met and she stared at me. Her eyes were wide and blue, so blue that they reminded me of someone— though I wasn't sure who. She smiled, and her teeth flashed white in my office. Her smile spread through the space between us, and I smiled back at her.

"So you're the doctor," she said.

It was more an accusation than an acknowledgment. Louise Billings raised her right arm and pointed her long thin finger toward me. "Little do you know," she said. "Little do you know."

The old woman shook her finger at me, wagging it back and forth in the air. I looked down at the pale white of her knuckles shining through the translucent skin, and then beyond that—I looked up into her blue eyes that shone out into the room. Deep down in her eyes I saw something bright and shiny, though I couldn't make out what it was.

A familiar smell came over me—a smell of soap and detergent and cleaning sprays, burning into my eyes and nose. I blinked and looked again into the old woman's eyes, and suddenly I was a child again, staring into the eyes of my aunt. I was standing with my father in the Caring Arms nursing home, carried back through time in the waters of my memory.

The woman I called "Annana" stopped shaking her hand back and forth. She pointed her thin, bony finger straight at me, and I saw her mouth open slowly and her teeth appear white and huge at the other end of her impossibly long arm. Behind me, I felt my father's hands press into my shoulders as the old woman spoke: "Little do you know," she said. "Little do you know."

The words were loud and clear and strong, and for an instant, all motion stopped in the room and there we were, only my aunt and I staring into each other's eyes.

"Doctor? Doctor? What does she mean?"

I heard the words softly, as if coming from a long ways away. My aunt's face shimmered and softened.

"What does she mean?"

I felt a hand on my arm, shaking it back and forth, and I blinked once more. My aunt's face faded, becoming dimmer and dimmer, until it vanished—replaced by the face of Louise Billings, who now sat smiling in front of me. Next to Louise, her granddaughter, June, leaned forward. "Doctor, are you all right?" she asked.

I looked from June's face to her grandmother, and back again. "I'm fine," I said. "Fine."

"She keeps repeating those words over and over," June said. "What do you think she means?"

I looked from June's young, worried frown to Louise Billings's smile. And I thought about all of the things doctors tell patients and their families. None of it made any sense to me just then. "I think your grandmother is right," I said.

"We know very little about this illness she has. We're still searching for its cause, still looking for a good treatment."

"Can't you do something?" June asked in a pleading tone.

She waited for my answer.

"I can be with you," I finally said. "I can listen."

Questions buzz around the edges of Alzheimer's disease, tiny sounds growing larger and larger until they fill my thoughts like flies that can't find an open window. "What do you think she means, Doctor? I know she recognizes me. She's trying to tell me something!"

Question after question. The sound grows larger, as if I had swatted at the flies and missed. It enters my head, buzzing, buzzing, and I know there must be a meaning to the questions. A meaning to Alzheimer's disease.

But what? There is no single answer, of course. And as I think about it, I close my eyes and my patients appear as real as if they were standing right next to me in the room.

There are the bent human beings, restrained in their wheelchairs and murmuring words that don't make sense into the air around them. The wanderers in the night, lost in their own neighborhoods as the cold winds come over them. And the men who, as their memories fail, awake to believe that their wives are not really their wives, but impostors who have stolen into their homes.

But there is more than this. There is Mario bursting into song at the nursing station, and Bridget dancing through my office; Samuel Ford criticizing Monet, and Laura Sunday bringing her sons together in the midst of her illness. There is Dr. Merlin at the lectern, Lawrence McGlynn surrounded by his memories of bright sunlight in Cuba, and Mona Lokal waking as if from a dream back into her life.

The meaning of Alzheimer's disease is found in my patients' lives. By their losses—of memory, direction, even language—they draw out a rough picture of the value of life, complete with all of its ragged edges. And even more important, by what they preserve—humor, hope, tears—my patients show me the persistent nature of life when it comes under siege.

These people touch me, and I am moved to examine the pieces of life that I am shown. As I write, I can see Louise's face as if she were sitting directly across from me in the room.

"Little do you know. Little do you know."

The words echo in my mind, and I know that they are true. I know very little about this illness of Alzheimer's disease, and I am humbled by it. But I learn more each day. I learn from sitting with my patients and their families and listening—listening and trying to hear—what it is they have to say.

Epilogue

I am reading a *New York Times* article on the current state of research and treatment of Alzheimer's disease. The basic premise of the piece is that although a great deal has been discovered about this illness in the past twenty years, and theories as to its cause abound, very little has changed in terms of the effects that physicians can have on the lives of their patients suffering from Alzheimer's.

Where *is* the hope in this illness? I spend the greatest part of my days with my patients and their families—listening to them, talking with them, trying to hold out a piece of the future for them to see that is not all dark and void of light.

We know far more now than we did twenty years ago. Geneticists have discovered rare mutations on chromosomes 1, 14, and 21 which can cause an uncommon type of Alzheimer's disease in families that occurs before the age of sixty. And we know that people with Down's syndrome (trisomy of chromosome 21) commonly develop Alzheimer's in midlife.

Perhaps some of the most exciting work has been done in the realm of genetic subtypes of apolipoproteins (apo)— molecules responsible for the transport of lipids in the brain. The gene for this molecule is on chromosome 19. Three different subtypes of the apolipoprotein type E gene are inherited: apo E2, apo E3, and apo E4.

Inheritance of the apo E4 subtype is a genetic risk factor for Alzheimer's disease. People with one copy of apo E4 are twice as likely to develop Alzheimer's, and people who have two copies of the apo E4 gene are up to eight times as likely to come down with the illness. But these people with apo E4 genes make up only a minority of the elderly.

Genetics is not the only arena in which theories of the cause of Alzheimer's exist. Many factors have been considered—nerve growth factors, hormonal factors, and neuroimmunological mechanisms are being investigated. There are theories of neuronal damage via steroids, inflammation, and oxidation. Some researchers even believe there is a role for programmed cell death eventually leading to Alzheimer's disease. And recently, there has been evidence that estrogen provides some protection against Alzheimer's.

But we do not know the cause of the illness. We don't know what causes the disease, and the mystery of not knowing is a painful thing for my patients and their families.

I keep staring at the *New York Times* article until the words blur and I remember Dori Sails.

Dori was the daughter of Frank Sails, an elderly man whom I saw one day in a nursing home consultation. Frank had been sent to live in the nursing home when his memory failed to the point where he couldn't take care of himself at home. All of the tests had been done, and no reversible cause had been found for Frank Sails's loss of memory. But it wasn't Frank Sails I remembered; it was his daughter, Dori.

"Don't you have a test that will diagnose this Alzheimer's?" she asked.

It was our first meeting, and I had just finished explaining to her that her father's history fit with a probable diagnosis of Alzheimer's disease.

"What do you mean 'probable'?" she asked. "Don't you know?"

Dori wanted an answer to her questions, and she found it very hard to accept the one I was giving her. She wanted something more definite than this. The next time I saw her was at the nursing home, several weeks later. I was entering her father's room when she came up behind me and took hold of my arm, steering me away from the door.

"Dr. Mathiasen, can I talk to you for a minute?"

Her hand tightened down on my forearm, and I looked up into the dark skin of her face. She had been crying. We walked over to a reception area near the entrance to the nursing home, and I sat down across from her. Dori started right in. "I have this terrible dream," she said, "and it keeps coming back every night."

Dori Sails's words came out in short, stuttering sentences between her tears. She told me that she was having a recurring nightmare of being stranded on a distant planet with her father. It had started the day after I first talked with her in the nursing home about his condition.

Dori had gone to bed and the dream had come over her as soon as she fell asleep. It was not a frightening dream at first. She and her father had just arrived on the planet—a world very much like earth. All of her friends lived there, people had the same jobs as they did here on earth, and life went on in much the same way. But there was one important difference. "This planet, this world, was slowly moving—being pulled, really— toward this huge black hole in space," Dori said.

Dori and her father had arrived on a world that was doomed, and they could not leave. She told me that they had flown there in a small spacecraft, and now she could not get the craft to fly again. They were trapped on the planet.

Everyone went about their lives exactly as they did on earth. But underneath the surface of this life, there was a sense of impending doom that spread out and infiltrated everything around her. This world was slowly moving toward a gaping black maw of space, and there was nothing anyone could do about it.

Each night, Dori would wake from the dream with her heart pounding, and several minutes would pass before she could stop shaking. The sense of doom that had invaded her dream stayed with her in her waking hours now. It would not fade.

"What do you think it means?" she asked me.

I didn't know what her dream meant, but as I looked into her open face I knew that I had to say something. "What does it mean to you, Dori?" I asked.

There was a long pause as Dori looked up into my face, as if searching for something. When she spoke again, it was in a low, soft voice. "I've been thinking about that a lot," she said.

Dori Sails told me that she knew the dream was symbolic, but it wasn't clear to her what it symbolized. The dream was exactly the same each night—she and her father were stranded on this distant planet, and they both wanted, more than anything else, to return to earth. But no matter what she did, she could not fix the spacecraft and get it to fly.

She kept coming back to the black hole in space, and the steady pull that she felt toward it. "No one seems concerned," she said. "They are all slowly drifting toward this oblivion, and no one is worried about it."

"Maybe they don't know it's happening," I said.

As soon as I finished the sentence, I could tell that I had

touched on something powerful in Dori's thoughts. Her hands dropped to her sides, and she looked like the wind had been knocked out of her. She told me that she had never even considered this, that she had assumed that everyone on the planet was aware of their impending doom, just as she was. But, she admitted, she had never asked anyone in the dream.

It occurred to me that Dori had not talked about her father's reaction to all of this either. I asked her how he acted in the dream. Her answer came back immediately: "He's scared of the black hole too, but we don't talk about it at all."

Dori Sails wasn't sure why she didn't talk to her father about their predicament in the dream. She told me that she hadn't even considered it. I asked Dori what her relationship with her father had been like in her adult life.

Frank Sails had been a very successful man in the construction business, and he had been away from home a great deal of the time while Dori was growing up. He loved her, and she knew it, but it was not something her father could put into words. Frank Sails had a need to be in control of all things in his life: his business dealings, his relationships, and above all, his emotions. To see him now, with his memory failing to the point where he could become lost in the nursing home, was very painful.

And then it came over me, and I thought that I understood Dori Sails's dream of a doomed planet.

There is no cure for Alzheimer's disease at the time of this writing. It slowly robs its sufferers of their memory, their thoughts, and eventually their reason as it moves through their lives. For those close to the one with Alzheimer's the disease is, in Nancy Reagan's eloquent phrase, "the long good-bye."

But we can treat the illness. Many of its symptoms respond to environmental changes. Over and over again I have seen the power of providing patients in the early stages of Alzheimer's disease with the opportunity to attend support groups and day-care centers. And as they progress further out into the disease, I can help their families make the decision on when the sufferer can no longer live at home.

Then there are the medical interventions. Many patients with Alzheimer's disease encounter complications because of the side effects of the medications they are taking. I don't mean only their psychiatric medications, but also the cardiac medicines, the antihypertensives, the pills for glaucoma and incontinence, and the blood thinners and all the rest that can cause problems.

People with Alzheimer's disease are much more vulnerable to becoming confused from the effects of too many medications, which can interact with one another and build up in their bloodstreams. As a rule, older people metabolize medications more slowly than they did when they were younger. Often, they appear as if their Alzheimer's is progressing rapidly, when in reality their increased confusion is being caused by too much medication.

Many patients improve dramatically when I stop a number of their prescriptions. They become more alert, more focused, and they feel better. This is always worth considering in Alzheimer's disease.

This brings us to the pharmacological treatment of Alzheimer's disease. There are many agents available for the treatment of complications of the illness: antidepressants, neuroleptics (e.g., Haldol, Trilafon, Risperdal), sedative-hypnotics, Buspar, lithium, sodium valproate, carbamazepine, and propranolol. The list goes on.

There is some evidence that the drug tacrine is effective in improving a patient's memory and intellectual function in the early stages of Alzheimer's disease, but the evidence is not very dramatic. And there are other agents, soon to appear on the U.S. market, with mechanisms of action similar to tacrine. They can at best slow down the progression of the illness. They cannot stop it.

The research goes on, but any cure for Alzheimer's disease is decades away.

Dori Sails's dream was not of a different world, although this is how it seemed to her. It was a dream of her own world and what it had become—a growing awareness of the pain and doubt that had invaded her father's life and then spread out into her life as well.

The uncertainty of her father's illness had become a part of her. The black hole in space was the black hole of Alzheimer's disease, and it pulled her in her sleep slowly down into a dark part of her soul where it was hard to see any light.

On my last visit with Dori and her father, I pulled her aside and told her my interpretation of the dream. As I finished, her mouth came open slightly and I saw the flash of white teeth in her dark face. "My God," she said slowly. Then she reached up with her hand and covered her mouth as she started to cry.

Dori Sails understood what I meant immediately. There are no right answers in the realm of dreams, but my words made sense to her. The dream was trying to tell her something—she knew that. And once she began to think of it as a revelation of what her world had become, then the fear and the sense of doom that she felt made sense. All of the people around her in the dream went about their lives, unaware of the sudden rent in the fabric of their existence that something like Alzheimer's disease could produce.

But Dori wanted more than understanding. She wanted to know how to help her father. "What can I do for him?" she asked me. "He is so alone."

Dori's question is the essential question in Alzheimer's disease: What can we do for the sufferer? It is one of the most difficult illnesses to deal with, because of the uncertainty that surrounds it. People usually live anywhere from six to eight years once the diagnosis is made, but they can live up to twenty years or more. Between the time of diagnosis and the end of life, there is a great deal of time. And it is important that this time is not lost.

I thought back to Dori Sails's question.

"Talk to your father about the dream," I told Dori.

She began to protest. "But he won't be able to understand me," she said. "He's too far gone—"

Dori stopped suddenly, covering her mouth with the palm of her hand as if to stop the flow of her words. She looked away, and her shoulders trembled as tears came into her eyes.

I told her again, quietly, that she should go to her father and talk to him about her dream. I told her that it was as much for her own benefit as for his, that it was an opportunity for her to draw closer to her father.

I don't think that Dori Sails believed me. But she did it anyway. She went into her father's room and told him about the dream of being stranded on a distant planet and falling slowly toward a black hole in space. I wasn't there for their talk. But one week later, I received a phone call from Dori.

"It stopped," she shouted into the phone. "The dream stopped."

Dori said that she sat down in her father's room at the nursing home that afternoon after she had talked with me, and although she felt foolish at first, she talked to her father about her dream. Just as she thought, he didn't seem to understand her words. But as she talked, she felt more relaxed and better than she had in a long time.

The afternoon stretched out, and she and her father talked about other things as well—family and friends and things that he could still understand. By the time she left the nursing home that day, she realized that it was the first time she and her father had tried to talk to each other in years and years. Then her bad dreams, and her sense of doom, came to an end.

This is Alzheimer's disease. In its fear and horror, lost among the plaques and tangles of the brain, is a force that can pull people together as well as push them apart. Until there is more certainty in the diagnosis and treatment of the illness, this is all that we have—the power of people talking and listening to one another, trying to understand the nature of their lives.

Index

213

Index

Index

listening, 13–14, 17, 20, 30, 78,
    87, 98, 201–2, 203
    refusal of, 166–67
Coumadin, 127, 128
Creutzfeldt-Jakob disease (CJD),
    37–38
Cuban baseball team, 110, 115–16,
    119, 121, 122–23, 127, 128–29
Curtiss, Dr. Jan, 124–25

day-care centers, 208
death:
    autopsies after, 80
    of brother, 49, 50, 52
    fear of, 24
    of the intellect, 79
    of spouse, 79–80, 83, 85, 94, 97
    waiting for, 24
dementia, 36, 97, 165–66
    and brain-wave patterns, 143
    diagnosis of, 169–70
    pseudo-dementia, 170
depression, 37, 183
    and Alzheimer-related fears,
        113–14, 115, 155
    anger in, 170
    and anxiety, 171
    diagnosis of, 81, 169–70, 185,
        186–87
    electroconvulsive therapy for,
        173, 174–81
    and hallucinations, 92–93
    and heredity, 173
    onset of, 171
    and physical problems, 170
    as pseudodementia, 170
    and PTSD, 71
    similarity to Alzheimer's, 81
    and suicide, 66, 173
diagnosis:
    differential, 80–81
    by elimination, 159
    history-based, 170

and passage of time, 42
and patient history, 80
technology and, 13, 38–42, 88,
    116–17, 123–25, 159–60
uncertainty of, 13, 25, 42, 63–64,
    80–81, 88, 112–14, 120, 126,
    127, 131–32, 143, 158–60,
    200–202, 204–5, 210, 211
differential diagnosis, 80–81
Dilantin, 127, 128
doctors:
    attacked by patients, 141–42
    blinded to emotional pain, 19,
        196
    bond of trust with, 78
    communication of patients and,
        13–15, 211
    in control, 141–42, 196
    effectiveness of, 203
    as medical students, 14
    moving patients along the assem-
        bly line, 18–19
    pressures on, 14, 64
    roles of, 34
dopamine, 92, 95, 97–101, 119
Down's syndrome, 201
dreams:
    and Alzheimer's, 195–96, 207,
        209–11
    PTSD nightmares, 70–71
    recurrent, 15–17, 195–96, 205–7
Dunner, Dr. Jake, 59, 60
dystonic reaction, 100–101

echocardiograms, McGlynn,
    124–25, 128
EEGs (electroencephalograms):
    Ford, 143–45
    McNamara, 59
    Merlin, 38
    Russolini, 155
EKGs (electrocardiograms),
    McGlynn, 123–25, 126

Index

electroconvulsive therapy, 173,
174–81
  bilateral vs. unilateral setting for,
  178
  discovery of, 174
  fear of, 175
  muscle-paralyzing drug and, 175,
  178, 179–80
  physical reactions to, 174, 179–80
  procedure of, 176–80
  and recovery, 181–83
  and schizophrenia, 174
emotions, and physical illness, 170
environmental changes, 208
epilepsy, and seizures, 120–22, 126,
127, 174
estrogen, 204

face, expressionless, 65, 66, 93
families:
  closeness of, 25, 192, 194
  communicating with, 114–15,
  210–11
  compensations made by, 79–80
  conflicts in, 192
  decisions made by, 208
  diagnosis sought by, 60
  fear of loss of, 98
  help for, 131–32, 154
  listening to, 14, 98
  and patient's sense of reality,
  85–88
  questions from, 97, 201, 204–5,
  210
  support from, 88
fears:
  Alzheimer-related, 24, 33,
  113–15, 155, 195, 196–97,
  209–10
  of being left alone, 166
  of death, 24
  escape from, 85
  and hallucinations, 98

of losing control, 196
of losing our families, 98
of losing our minds, 24, 196
of shock treatment, 175
fibrillation, atrial, 123–26
Ford, Arthur, and brother's illness,
134–37, 146–50
Ford, Samuel, 133–50
  in adult family home, 148
  as art collector, 135, 137–38,
  149–50
  charisma of, 148, 149
  confusion of, 134–35, 137, 139,
  143, 148
  diagnosis of, 143
  electronic journal of, 133–34,
  138–39
  family background of, 137–38
  memory loss of, 138
  monitoring of, 144–45
  seizures of, 135–36, 139, 140–43,
  145–48
  treatment of, 139, 143, 147
  violence of, 136, 139–43, 144–46,
  147–48
forgetting, fear of, 24, 33
Freud, Sigmund, 170
Friedman, Dr. Arthur, 91–93
friends and families, *see* families

genetics, 203–4
geriatric psychiatry, 18, 19, 20
grand mal seizures, 120–22, 126
  anticonvulsant medication for,
  127
  and electroconvulsive therapy,
  174

Haldol, 95, 99–100, 103, 118
hallucinations:
  and Alzheimer's, 108, 112, 115,
  118
  and blood clots, 126

Index

and brain, 92–93, 95, 97, 115,
   116, 117, 119
   of N. Brown, 63, 67, 73–74
   causes of, 115–18, 119–20, 126
   and depression, 92–93
   and fears, 98
   and infections, 115
   of L. McGlynn, 107–12, 115,
      116–23, 127–29
   and medication, 94–95, 99,
      103–4, 115, 118–19
   and psychoses, 102, 103
   of B. Texas, 105–6
   of O. Texas, 92–99, 101–2, 103–5
heart:
   atrial fibrillation of, 123–26
   blood clots in, 124, 125–26, 128
   echocardiograms of, 124–25, 128
   EKG of, 123–25, 126
   electrical impulses in, 124
heredity:
   and Alzheimer's, 196–97, 198
   and depression, 173
hormonal factors, 204
Huntington's chorea, 92

infections:
   and hallucinations, 115
   and spinal taps, 155
inflammation, 204

judgment, lapses of, 80

Kahn, Dr. Larry, 50
Kubota, Dr. Al, 63, 67, 72, 73, 76–77
kuru, 37–38

language:
   breaking apart of, 27, 37
   facility in, 108, 114–15
   word recall, 80, 114
levodopa, 93, 168
life, value of, 202

life force, 132, 168, 202
Lifeline, senior citizen complex, 49,
   50, 52–53, 57, 60–61
listening:
   to family and friends, 14, 98
   to ghosts under the surface, 17
   to patients, 13–14, 17, 20, 30, 78,
      87, 201–2, 203
   psychiatry and, 15
   and slowing down, 20
liver, and Tylenol, 33–34
Lokal, Mona, 165–83
   dementia of, 165–70
   depression of, 169, 170, 171–73
   diagnosis of, 165–66, 169–70
   first visit with, 166–69
   not communicating, 166–67
   not eating, 166, 173
   in nursing home, 165, 169, 172
   recovery of, 181–83
   shock treatments of, 173, 174–81
Lokal, Shirley, and mother's illness,
   166, 170–72, 175–76, 182–83

McGlynn, Karen, and husband's illness, 107–22, 125–29
McGlynn, Lawrence, 107–29, 132
   atrial fibrillation of, 123–26
   and Cuban baseball team, 110,
      115–16, 119, 121, 122–23,
      127, 128–29
   depression of, 113–14
   echocardiograms of, 124–25, 128
   EKG of, 123–25, 126
   first wife of, 111
   forgetfulness of, 113–14
   grand mal seizures of, 120–22,
      126, 127
   hallucinations of, 107–12, 115,
      116–23, 127–29
   language facility of, 108, 114–15
   medication of, 118–19, 127–28
   MRI of, 116, 117, 123, 126–27

217

Index

Index

Index

Index